The History of Plastic Surgery

THE HISTORY OF

PLASTIC SURGERY

From the Collection of

Douglas M. Monasebian, M.D., D.M.D., F.A.C.S.

An Exhibition Held at the Grolier Club

November 19, 2020 – February 13, 2021

The Grolier Club
New York
2020

CONTENTS

PREFACE

I AM NOT SURE if every historian is a bibliophile, but I am quite sure that every bibliophile is a historian. To collect books not only requires one to understand the world as it was when the book was written but to appreciate the thoughts and ideas of the author as he went about his writings. As my personal collection grew, this became my driving force. I sought out books in plastic surgery that not only had significance in the progression of plastic surgery as a medical discipline but also possessed historical importance. Studies on facial expression, disease, and obesity were just as interesting to me as the first surgical descriptions of nasal reconstruction or cleft palate repair were. While I have not always collected the aforementioned books, being a passionate collector has been a significant part of my life from a young age. At eight years old, I began collecting baseball cards; my collecting interest then shifted to *Mad* magazine through adolescence. I also recognized as a child that I wanted to become a surgeon. I was fascinated by science, loved working with my hands, but most importantly desired to be in a profession where I could help people. After graduating from dental school, I had a thirst for more knowledge in a different field of work and continued my education by going to medical school. I completed residencies in both oral and maxillofacial surgery and plastic surgery and then ventured into private practice. As I grew comfortable in my private practice and had more discretionary time, I studied more on the history of my profession and learned that the fathers of modern-day plastic surgery were trained in the same fashion as myself. Their entry into this type of work was for different reasons; however, that made little difference to me. These individuals had medical and dental backgrounds and focused primarily on facial reconstructions that became increasingly prevalent because of the injuries soldiers suffered during World War I. This unique history enriched my experience and inspired me in my profession, which culminated in a desire to learn even more about the specialty. As with most surgeons, I can be obsessively compulsive and love to face different challenges. My new goal became to learn from everything I could get my hands on to uncover the multifaceted and fabulous history of plastic surgery. Unlike my past collecting endeavors, there is no simple checklist applicable here. One does not and cannot acquire sequential cards or magazine numbers and deem the collection to be complete. As any true collector knows, the deeper one gets into the collection, the further it spreads out. I saw myself seeking out not only books but photographs, autographed letters, instruments, and paper ephemera. All of it found a place in the collection and complemented the whole beautifully.

As medicine evolved throughout the last millennium, so did surgery. The barber surgeons of the sixteenth and seventeenth centuries were becoming more daring and sophisticated in their approaches to surgery. Although crude for the modern-day, some plastic surgery procedures have withstood the test of time and are still successfully employed today. For example, Tagliacozzi's forehead flap can still be used, as can skin-grafting practices from the 1800s. The advent of antisepsis, anesthesia, and asepsis in the nineteenth century helped to make plastic surgery safer and more predictable. To the contrary, cleft lip repairs prior to the eighteenth century are now outdated.

I trust your exploration of this exhibit will allow you to share in the joy I have had while creating it. I also want to take this opportunity to thank my beloved parents, who continually inspired me to "do whatever I wanted to do in life, as long as it was to the best of my best ability." And to my beautiful wife and children, thank you for your patience and support as my collection grew and diversified.

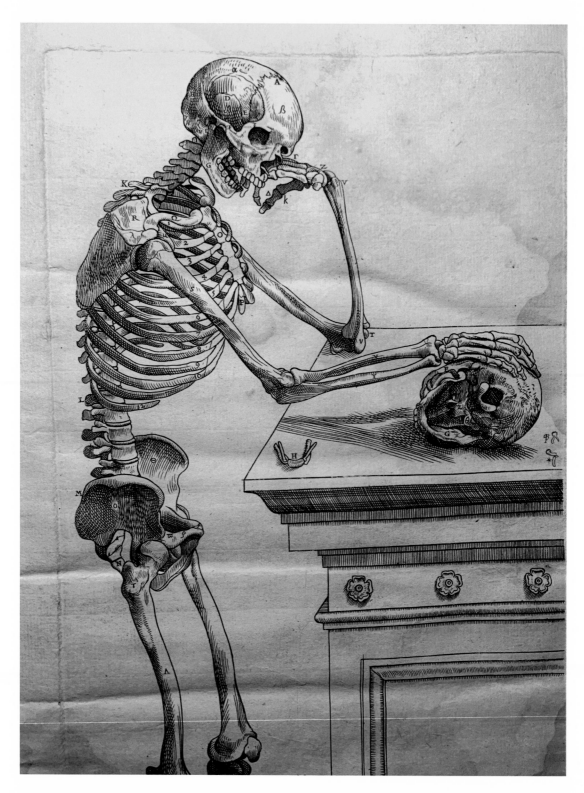

No. 1.

The Dawn of Plastic Surgery

The modern definition of plastic surgery is rooted in ancient medicine. The Sanskrit text *Sushruta Samhita*, written around 600 BC by the ancient Indian medical practitioner Sushruta, describes the quintessential plastic surgery procedure of a nasal reconstruction utilizing tissue harvested from the cheek. During the sixteenth century, Italian surgeon Gaspare Tagliacozzi and French surgeon Ambrose Paré adopted these early procedures and started to use local and distant tissue to reconstruct complex wounds. Further advances in similar procedures were made by prominent European plastic surgeons in the eighteenth and nineteenth centuries. For example, in the nineteenth century, German surgeon Karl Ferdinand von Gräfe first used the term *plastic* when describing creative reconstructions of the nose. The term *plastic surgery* stems from the Greek word *plastikos*, meaning "to mold" or "to form." Today, plastic surgery can be broadly defined as the functional, structural, and aesthetic restoration of all manner of defects and deformities of the human body. Modern plastic surgery has evolved into the two broad categories of reconstructive and aesthetic surgery. Reconstructive plastic surgery aims to restore the normal condition, and aesthetic surgery strives to improve the normal condition. Prior to the early twentieth century, almost all plastic surgery was reconstructive in nature. Following World War I, advancements were made in both facial reconstruction and facial aesthetic surgery, which allowed the specialty to evolve and progress given technological and educational developments. Aesthetic, or cosmetic, surgery became more accepted, and, as advancements were made, surgery also became safer and less invasive. Additionally, cosmetic surgery began to be performed on the breasts and body.

1. ℂ THOMAS GEMINUS. *Compendiosa Totius Anatomie Delineatio* [A complete delineation of the entire anatomy]. London: John Herford, 1545.

Thomas Geminus (Thomas Lambert or Lambrit), an engraver, mathematician, and surgical instrument maker, published this book as an abridged and pirated copy of Vesalius's *Fabrica*, originally published in 1543. It is illustrated with figures from both Vesalius's *Fabrica* and *Epitome* and re-engraved in copperplate. The book was dedicated to Henry VIII who, five years earlier, had given assent to an act uniting the barbers' and surgeons' guilds. Later that same year, another act supplied cadavers to the newly formed Company of Barbers and Surgeons for dissection. This work would help provide greatly needed anatomical information to members of that guild.

2. ℂ AULUS CORNELIUS CELSUS. *De Medicina* [On medicine]. Basel: Johannes Oporinus, 1552.

Aulus (or Aurelius) Cornelius Celsus, an encyclopedist and possibly a practicing physician, wrote this encyclopedic book drawing upon the ancient Greeks. The work was first published in the first century and was the earliest complete text to follow the tripartite division of medicine as established by Hippocrates and Asclepiades: diet, pharmacology, and surgery. His work espouses advanced medical practices urging cleanliness and antisepsis, using vinegar and thyme oil. He also discusses reconstructive plastic surgery of the face utilizing tissue and skin from other parts of the body. Using such tissue flaps is still practiced today.

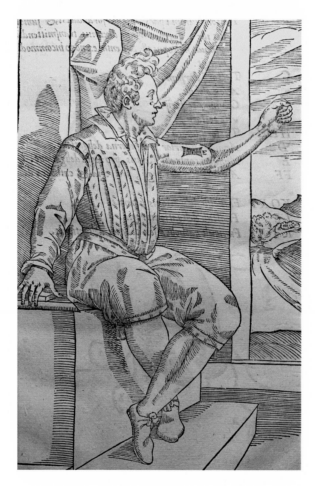

No. 3.

3. ℭ GASPARE TAGLIACOZZI. *De Curtorum Chirurgia per Insitionem* [On the surgery of mutilation by grafting]. Venice: Gaspare Bindoni the younger, 1597.

Gaspare Tagliacozzi, both a philosopher and a physician, was well known throughout Europe outside his native Bologna. This work built upon those of distant predecessors such as Celsus and the more recent Gustavo Branca of Sicily. The *De Curtorum* is the first book exclusively devoted to plastic surgery. Tagliacozzi discusses the "Italian Method" of nasal reconstruction involving a delayed flap from the forehead skin, thoroughly considering every aspect of the flap from design to postoperative care. A quotation from his book has become a standard of care in plastic surgery to this day: *"We restore, rebuild, and make whole those parts which nature hath given, but which fortune has taken away. Not so much that it may delight the eye, but that it might buoy up the spirit, and help the mind of the afflicted."*

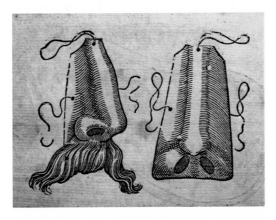

No. 4.

4. ℂ AMBROSE PARÉ. *Les œuvres* [The works]. London: John Clarke, 1665.

Ambrose Paré, a French barber surgeon, is considered to be a father of both surgery and forensic pathology. This comprehensive work discusses many facets of surgery of that era. Particularly known for his work on battlefield medicine and the treatment of war wounds, Paré also reintroduced Galen's method of artery ligation instead of heat cauterization, the latter often failing as a means to cease bleeding during amputations. Paré also made numerous contributions to rehabilitation with his work on limb prostheses following amputation, as well as ocular prostheses fashioned from gold, silver, porcelain, and glass. Unlike others in reconstructive nasal surgery, he favored a nasal prosthesis over autogenous tissue reconstruction.

5. ℂ ROGER BACON. *The Cure of Old Age and Preservation of Youth.* Translated from the Latin by Richard Browne. London: Thomas Flesher, 1683.

Roger Bacon (also known as Frater Rogerus or Doctor Mirabilis) was a philosopher and Franciscan friar known for his study of nature through empiricism. In this book, Bacon teaches ways to cure illness and keep off the accidents of old age while preserving the youth, beauty, and strength of the body. He recognized the connection between a sound mind and a sound body. Although surgical rejuvenation of the body was not possible then, Bacon espoused many other ways to preserve youth. It would take over two centuries until surgeons started to develop surgical means for rejuvenation.

6. ℂ GEORGE II. *Surgeons and Barbers of London Act, 1741.* London: Thomas Baskett, 1745.

The Black Plague wiped out the majority of physicians in the 14th and 15th centuries. This created a great demand for barbers and their surgical procedures. Coupling with that was the fact that universities during the Renaissance did not provide formal education in surgery because it was considered a trade due to its manual nature. Therefore, it was difficult to accept that surgeons were equal to medical doctors. Physicians trained together in medical school to earn their medical degree, while barber-surgeons trained as apprentices and sat for an exam to obtain their diploma. Today's surgical residency programs still follow this method. In the 1540s, barbers and surgeons joined together to form the United Company of Barbers and Surgeons in order to gain credibility. Their combined guild lasted for over two hundred years. In 1745 the surgeons broke away from the barbers to form the Company of Surgeons, which became the Royal College of Surgeons in 1800. This proclamation separating the combined guild into two separate guilds was printed by Thomas Baskett, the son of John Baskett, the official printer to the King.

7. ℂ WILLIAM HOGARTH. *The Analysis of Beauty*. London: John Reeves, 1753.

William Hogarth was an English satirist and editorial cartoonist, as well as a painter and print-maker. In *The Analysis of Beauty*, Hogarth discusses the six principles that he felt affect and influence beauty. He admits that these principles have an effect, but he does not commit to each of their influences. The principles are fitness, variety, regularity, simplicity, intricacy, and quantity. His principles served to formulate an objective basis to beauty that still holds true today. This work serves as a useful adjunct to Roger Bacon's work on the cure for old age.

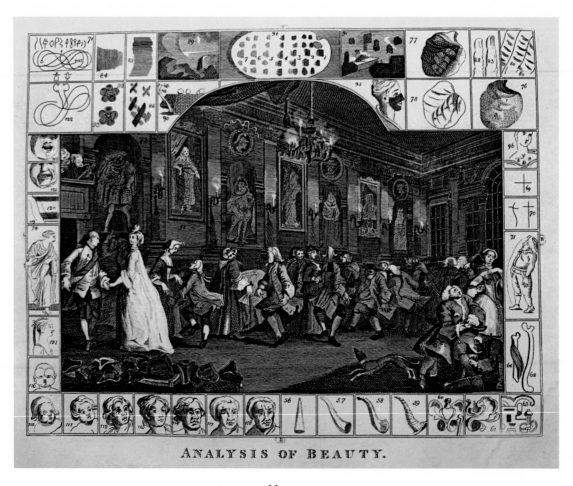

No. 7.

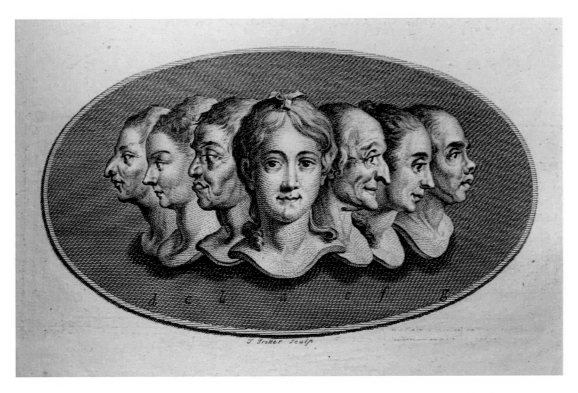

No. 8.

8. ℂ JOHANN KASPAR LAVATER. "Of the Harmony between Moral Beauty and Physical Beauty." In *Essays on Physiognomy*. Vol. 1. London: John Murray, 1789.

Johann Kaspar Lavater was a Protestant pastor and Swiss writer. The word physiognomy is derived from the Greek *physis*, meaning "nature," and *gnomon*, meaning "judge" or "interpreter." Physiognomy involves the art of assessing one's character or personality from his or her outer appearance and expression, especially the face. The term also refers to the general appearance of a person or object. Physiognomy dates back to ancient times with the poets of Greece and the Siddhars of India. Ancient Chinese practiced mianxiang, or "face reading." Aristotle and Zopyrus were also known to practice ancient physiognomy. Lavater is credited for promoting modern physiognomy. His *Essays on Physiognomy*, originally published in German, were later translated into French and English.

9. ℂ CHARLES BELL. *Illustrations of the Great Operations of Surgery*. London: Longman, Hurst, Rees, Orme and Brown, 1821.

Charles Bell was a noted Scottish surgeon and anatomist of the early 19th century. Most noted for describing Bell's palsy, he also discovered the differences between sensory and motor nerves in the spinal cord. His *Great Operations* meticulously details the sentinel operations in surgery, including hernia repair, amputation, and aneurism repair. The book includes twenty etched plates by Thomas Landseer after drawings by Bell. Bell is also credited for writing the first works on the notions of the anatomy and physiology of facial expression for illustrators and painters in 1806.

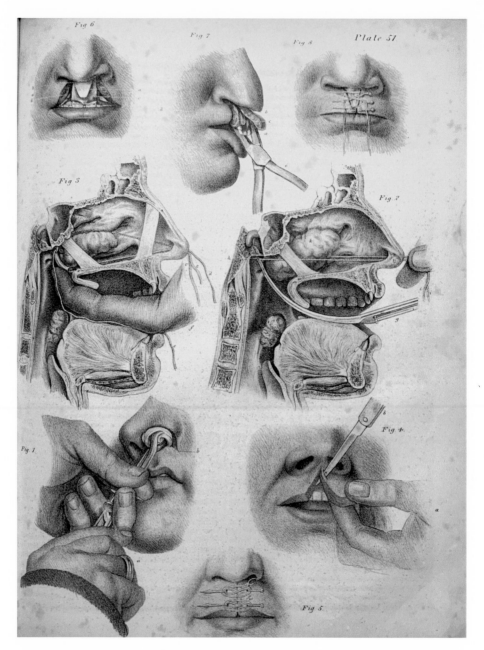

No. 12.

10. ¶ Phillippe-Frédéric Blandin. *Autoplastie* [Autoplasty]. Paris: d'Urtubie et Worms, 1836.

Phillippe-Frédéric Blandin was a French Surgeon of the mid-19th century who worked as an anatomical assistant to the faculty of medicine in Paris, where he later became a prosector (one who prepares a body for dissection for demonstration purposes). Although well known in the field of plastic surgery for his work on rhinoplasty, he is best known for his work on autoplasty, which is the surgical procedure of taking tissue form one body part and transferring it to another for reconstructive purposes. This procedure, which is still employed today, served as the basis for many other future reconstructive plastic surgical procedures.

11. ℭ FRIEDRICH AUGUST VON AMMON. *Die plastiche Chirurgie* [Plastic surgery]. Berlin: Verlag von G. Reimer, 1842.

Friedrich August von Ammon was a German surgeon specializing in ophthalmology. He settled in Dresden, Germany, and was known for his works in ophthalmology and plastic surgery; he was also responsible for helping to develop each one into a separate specialty. He developed procedures in oculoplastic surgery and penned a prize-winning book on eyelid surgery. His work on plastic surgery was the first to survey the entire history of plastic surgery.

12. ℭ JOSEPH PANCOAST. *A Treatise on Operative Surgery*. Philadelphia: Carey and Hart, 1844.

Joseph Pancoast was an America surgeon responsible for many of the sentinel advances in surgery. He not only described these procedures but published graphic depictions of them as well. His treatise is his greatest work, containing over four hundred eighty illustrations with over eighty plates. His contributions to plastic surgery within the book include the formation of a nose by means of plough and groove, an eyebrow reconstruction with a transposed scalp flap, and turndown flaps of abdominal skin for bladder exstrophy treatment. His abdominal tourniquet, which compressed the aorta, saved many lives during procedures invloving increased blood loss such as lower extremity amputation.

13. ℭ HEINRICH VON PFOLSPREUNDT. *Buch der Béndth-Ertznei* [Book of the Béndth-Ertznei]. Berlin: Druck and Verlag von G. Reimer, 1868.

Heinrich von Pfolspreundt (or Pfolsprundt) was a German army surgeon. He advanced medical and surgical practice during the late medieval and early Renaissance periods. This work, originally written in 1460 but not published until 1868, served to advance the practice of medicine and surgery. The book discusses military surgery and alludes to the removal of bullets and treatment of war injuries. It includes one of the earlier accounts of Western rhinoplasty after Celsus and, more recently, the Brancas from Sicily. He also proposed suturing techniques for the repair of a cleft lip, a technique more anatomic and functional than others performed during his time.

14. ℭ DAVID PRINCE. *Plastics and Orthopedics*. Philadelphia: Lindsay and Blakiston, 1871.

David Prince was an American surgeon, who served as brigade surgeon to the Army of the Potomac under General McClellan. When McClellan was forced to retreat, the patients within the hospital were captured. At first, Prince refused to be exchanged for another prisoner, but he later acquiesced and went back to Jacksonville, IL. He then built a hospital and took care of the wounded, where he perfected many procedures in both plastic surgery and orthopedic surgery. His Prince Infirmary treated over three thousand patients a year. Many of these treatments were in the field of plastic surgery, including burn procedures and cancer reconstructions. He was also a great proponent of antisepsis.

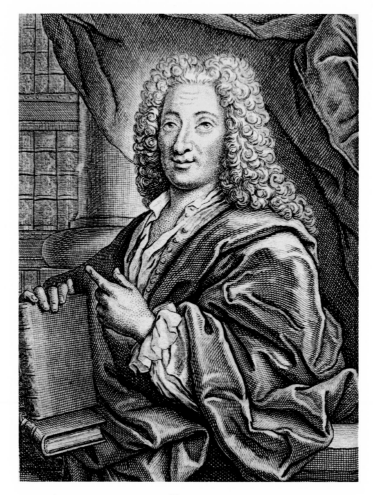

No. 15.

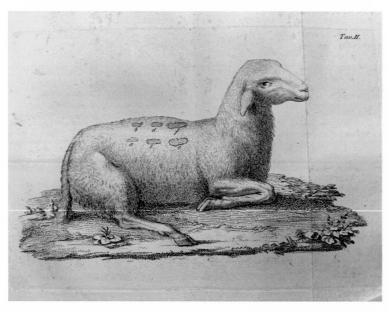

No. 16.

Illness and Disease

The main tenets of medicine include both accurate diagnosis and treatment. As surgeons, the practitioners of plastic surgery used what was available to them to restore the parts of the human body that were lost or ravished by illness, disease, trauma, or birth defect. The guiding principles of restoration of form and function were as important hundreds of years ago as they are today. Medical anatomy was also beginning to be formally described, which helped these early surgeons advance in their practice of surgery and perform plastic surgery on all parts of the body and on all age groups. This advance included skin grafting, which entailed transplanting pieces of skin from one part of the body to another without a blood supply. Tissue flaps were also being performed, which transferred adjacent segments of skin and muscle with an attached blood supply to restore and fill those aforementioned lost defects. Plastic surgeons adapted well, not only utilizing what was available to them at the time but constantly forging forward in their thinking, planning, and ultimate execution. What made these advancements possible, of course, was concurrent medical progress in anesthesia, antisepsis, and instrumentation. Today an entire face with its attached skin, muscle, nerves, bone, and blood supply can be transplanted.

15. ⁋ PIERRE FAUCHARD. *Le chirurgien dentiste* [The surgeon dentist]. Paris: Chez Pierre-Jean Mariette, 1746.

Although trained as a physician, Pierre Fauchard is widely regarded as the father of modern dentistry. In *Le chirurgien dentiste*, Fauchard describes basic oral anatomy and function. He also discusses oral medicine and pathology as well as procedures for both the removal and restoration of teeth. He starts most of the book devoted to the care and treatment of the face and jaws in the specialty known today as oral and maxillofacial surgery—one of the precursors of modern-day plastic surgery. Fauchard is also credited for inventing and improving surgical instruments. He borrowed ideas for these fine instruments from the watchmakers and jewelers at the time. He even was inspired by the instruments and tools of the barbers. He was also known for the fabrication of dental prostheses for the replacement of teeth that were lost to extraction or disease.

16. ⁋ GIUSEPPE BARONIO. *Degli innesti animali* [On grafting in animals]. Milan: Dalla stamperia e fonderia del Genio, 1804.

Giuseppe Baronio was both a physician and a physiologist. In this book he recounts his experiments with skin transplantation on a sheep. This marked the beginning of skin grafting in plastic surgery. These skin grafts were carried out by the detachment of skin from one part of the body and transplanted to other parts, where they successfully healed. A successful take, or survival, of the graft was noted by the presence of hair growth. The research was conducted very scientifically and in a controlled manner. It took another thirteen years for the first successful skin grafting to be performed on humans.

17. ℭ WILLIAM WADD. *Comments of Corpulency*. London: John Ebers & Co., 1829.

William Wadd was not only a medical author but also a noted British surgeon. In his *Comments of Corpulency*, Wadd discusses through anecdote and experience not only the diseases of obesity but leanness and diet as well. He was one of the earlier advocates of a sensible approach to food. He concluded that obesity was simply a result of "an overindulgence at the table." His work was highly influential, and dieting consequently became more poplar during the Victorian era. Wadd was also a skilled artist and draftsman and is credited with the drawing of all the etchings in the book. Today, the Wadd Society is dedicated to the exploration of the history of obesity.

18. ℭ MAXIMILIAN JOSEPH CHELIUS. "Gelungene Lippen- und Nasenbildung" [Successful lips and nose formation]. In *Heidelberg Clinical Annals*. Vol. 6. Heidelberg: J. C. B. Mohr, 1830.

Maximilian Joseph Chelius was both a German surgeon and an ophthalmologist, who worked as a military surgeon in Munich. In this early treatise on plastic surgery, Chelius describes a reconstruction of the upper lip and nose utilizing a forehead flap. Known for his surgery on the head, neck, and eye, his most famous patient did not suffer from a head-and-neck ailment, but rather one who was treated for an infection of the finger. This patient was Frédéric Chopin. Chopin repaid Chelius by the performance of a private concert. Chelius was a catalyst in the development of the medical faculty at Heidelberg University and was considered the founder of the surgical tradition at that institution.

19. ℭ ALFRED VELPEAU. *Nouveaux éléments de médecine opératoire* [New elements of operative medicine]. 2 vols. Brussels: H. Dumont, 1832.

Alfred Velpeau was a French hospital surgeon. He was not only the most skilled surgeon in France during the first half of the 19th century but was also a master of anatomy. He authored hundreds of texts not only about surgery and anatomy but also in the fields of embryology and obstetrics. *Médecine opératoire* was the most detailed surgical work on France in the middle of the 19th century. In it, Velapeau describes and classifies numerous plastic surgical procedures. These include detailed procedures of face and breast reconstructions. An atlas with exquisite illustrations was also printed as a supplement.

20. ℭ JOHN HUNTER. *Hunterian Reminiscences*. London: Sherwood, Gilbert, and Piper, 1833.

John Hunter was a Scottish surgeon and one of the more distinguished and respected surgeons of his day. He was an early believer in the scientific method of medicine, which mandated careful observation. He gained an appreciation for anatomy by assisting his elder brother, William, at his anatomy school in London. He quickly became an expert in anatomy and spent years as a surgeon in the army. He amassed a collection of animals whose skeletons and other organs he

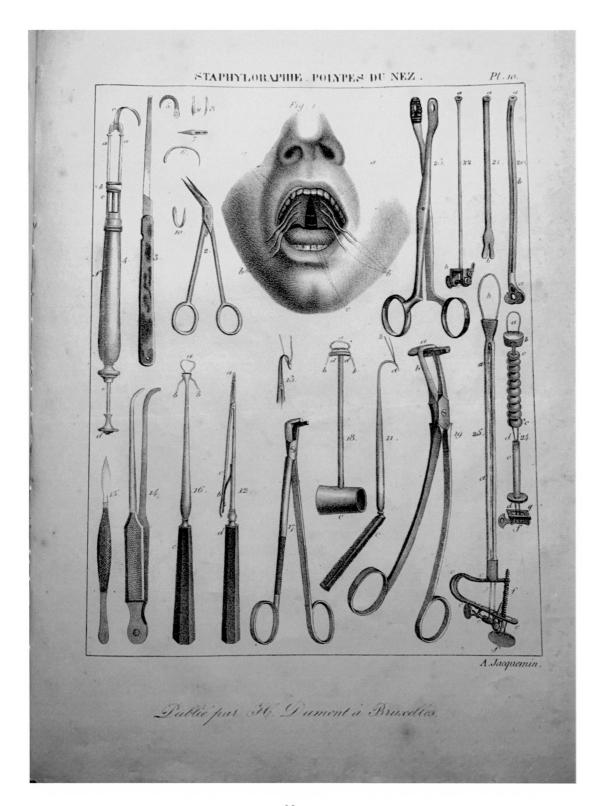

Fig. 1.

A. Jacquemin.

Publié par H. Dumont à Bruxelles.

No. 19.

prepared as anatomical specimens. He eventually amassed nearly 14,000 preparations demonstrating the anatomy of humans and other vertebrates, including over 3,000 animals. In his *Reminiscences*, Hunter discusses his lectures and principles in the practice of surgery. The Hunterian Society in London is named for him, as is the Hunterian Museum at the Royal College of Surgeons, which curates his collection of anatomical specimens.

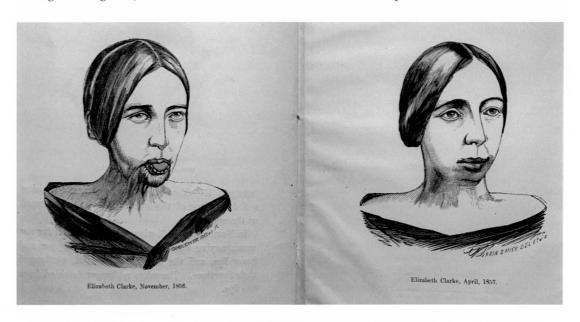

Elizabeth Clarke, November, 1856.

Elizabeth Clarke, April, 1857.

No. 21.

21. ℂ THOMAS TEALE. *On Plastic Operations for the Restoration of the Lower Lip.* London: John Churchill, 1857.

Thomas Teale was a British surgeon in the mid-19th century. He came from a family of surgeons and was a founder of the Leeds School of Medicine. The loss of one eye during his youth did not deter him. In this rare publication, Teale describes restorations of the lower lip (cheiloplasty) and reconstructions of other deformities of the face and neck. There is discussion of eyelid reconstruction as well. The surgical descriptions are accompanied by very fine illustrations.

22. ℂ CHRISTOPHER HEATH. *Injuries and Diseases of the Jaws.* London: John Churchill, 1868.

Christopher Heath was a British surgeon and anatomist. He was also proficient in dental surgery. The jaws are the solid foundation to the face, in which surgeons continued to have a keen interest. In this book, Heath discusses not only injuries and diseases of the jaws but of the antra and sinuses. The treatment of these maladies is discussed both surgically and medically. Heath also led a very didactic life, serving as an examiner in both surgery and dental surgery.

23. ℂ James Garretson. *A Treatise on the Diseases and Surgery of the Mouth, Jaws and Associated Parts.* Philadelphia: J. B. Lippincott, 1869.

James Garretson was an American surgeon and dentist in the mid-19th century. He taught at the oral surgery clinic at the Dental College of Pennsylvania. He was personally responsible for establishing the dental specialty of oral and maxillofacial surgery. He is aptly named the father of oral surgery. He used the first dental engine, or drill, for bone surgery and grafting. He devised techniques for the treatment of jaw fractures. In this book he discusses the diagnosis, management, and treatment of diseases of the oral cavity including the mouth and jaws. The treatise was written for both practitioners and students.

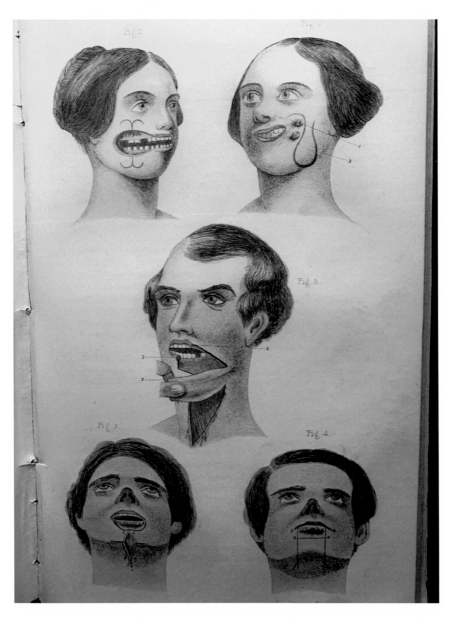

No. 23.

24. ℂ LOUIS OLLIER. "Greffes cutanées ou autoplastiques" [Cutaneous and auto-plastic transplants]. Bulletin de l'Académie de médecine 1, ser. 2 (1872).

Louis Ollier was a 19th-century French surgeon. Although famous for his work in bone and joint surgery, his greatest contributions to plastic surgery were in furthering the development of techniques in skin grafting, for which he is best known. In this work, Ollier reports devising thicker skin grafts and asserts that the recipient site should also be prepared adequately so as to accept the graft. Previously, this was not being done, leading to the failure of many skin grafts. He showed that these grafts, covering areas of tissue loss, allow faster healing and with a better quality scar. The term "skin graft" was coined by Ollier. He also declared that a skin graft should be used whenever a skin flap is not possible.

25. ℂ KARL THIERSCH. "Über die feineren anatomischen Veränderungen bei Auf-heilung von Haut auf Granulationen" [On the finer anatomical changes in healing of skin on granulations]. *Verhandlungen der Deutschen Gesell-schaft für Chirurgie* 3, no. 69 (1874).

Karl Thiersch was a 19th-century German surgeon who was also a noted anatomist. In this journal article, Thiersch builds upon Ollier's work, cutting free grafts of skin up to one centimeter in diameter. These were not the Thiersch grafts that were utilized later on, however. He was also a proponent of the concept of "flagellation," where the donor region (from where the skin is harvested) was traumatized in order to increase its survival when transplanted.

26. ℂ GURDON BUCK. *Contributions to Reparative Surgery.* New York: D. Appleton & Co., 1876.

Gurdon Buck was a pioneering 19th-century American military plastic surgeon during the Civil War. He is known for being the first doctor to incorporate pre-operative and post-operative photographs into his publications, a standard in today's plastic surgery environment. His first published, illustrated medical photograph was of a fused knee joint. This book on reparative surgery is considered the first American plastic surgery textbook essentially devoted to reconstructive surgery.

27. ℂ GEORGE FOX AND FREDERIC STRUGIS. *Medicine and Surgery: Illustrated.* New York: E. B. Treat, 1882.

George Fox and Fredric Strugis were American physicians of the late 19th century. In this profusely illustrated book and atlas, they discuss numerous illnesses of the human body, with an emphasis on the disease process and surgical treatments. The work also includes the plastic operation for the loss of the nose and eyelids; another chapter considers the restoration of the lip. In this atlas, they were the first authors to use the mechanical photographic printing process developed in 1878 known as the artotype.

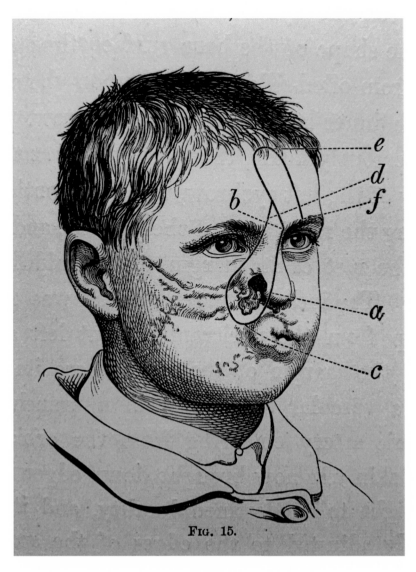

FIG. 15.

No. 26.

28. ℂ JOHN ROBERTS. *The Surgical Treatment of Disfigurement and Deformities of the Face.* Philadelphia: Philadelphia Medical Publishing Co., 1901.

John Roberts was an American surgeon in the late 19th and early 20th centuries. In addition to his work in facial surgery, he was a pioneering surgeon in cranial surgery. In this book he espouses many surgical techniques still in use today. He was a strong proponent of antisepsis in the field of neurosurgery. In addition to publishing works on neurosurgery, he wrote and edited books in general surgery, orthopedic surgery, and plastic surgery. In this book he discusses surgical management and treatment of facial injuries, particularly those caused from war wounds.

Nasal Reconstruction

The reconstruction of the nose dates back thousands of years, and the ancient Hindus are credited with the first nasal reconstruction attempts. In ancient India, punishment involved having one's nose cut off, and such a defect was reportedly first repaired by transposing a cheek flap. The Italians also executed reconstructive techniques for the nose during the Renaissance, when the Branca family and Tagliacozzi experimented with arm flaps and rhinoplasty techniques. Additionally, the British documented the Indian techniques of reconstruction they saw during their time in the subcontinent. Gillies, of England, formulated rules and techniques for nasal reconstruction as he helped those injured during wartime. These efforts were passed on, expanded, and refined to form the multitude of reconstructive options available today which not only include the aesthetic reconstruction of the nose, but the functioning of the nose as well. With the advent of cosmetic surgery at the turn of the twentieth century, rhinoplasty techniques branched out to cosmetic rhinoplasties as the demand for a more beautiful nose rose.

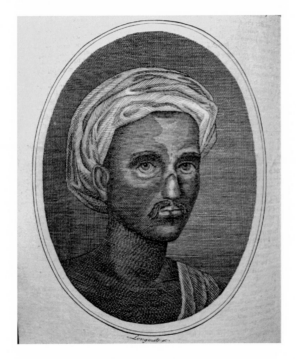

No. 29.

29. ⟨ B.L. "[Indian Rhinoplasty]." *Gentleman's Magazine* 64, pt.2, no. 4 (1794).

In this issue of *Gentleman's Magazine*, a reader identified as "B.L." reported on a nasal reconstruction performed in the then-British colony of India. This report revolutionized the practice of rhinoplasty, which had not been written about in nearly 200 years. This case study, written by a non-medical practitioner in a non-medical journal, describes a bullock driver named Cowassjee in the English army during the war of 1792, when he had his nose and arm chopped off while held as a prisoner at war. The reconstructed nose was made from a forehead flap as described by Tagliacozzi centuries prior. Although published for a popular readership, the report does show the stages of the reconstruction. This article helped to spark a revival of plastic surgical operations in the 19th century.

30. ⁋ JOSEPH CARPUE. *An Account of Two Successful Operations for Restoring a Lost Nose. . . .* London: Longman, Hurst, Rees, Orme and Brown, 1816.

Joseph Carpue was an English surgeon in the early 19th century. He is credited with the first nasal reconstruction in England, performing the surgery on the nose of an army officer whose nose collapsed from chronic mercury treatments for a disease of the liver. It was performed under no anesthetic, reportedly in less than thirty minutes, from forehead skin as described previously as the Italian method. Although he became famous for this rhinoplastic procedure, Carpue has also been credited for his experiments with electricity in medicine and their therapeutic benefits.

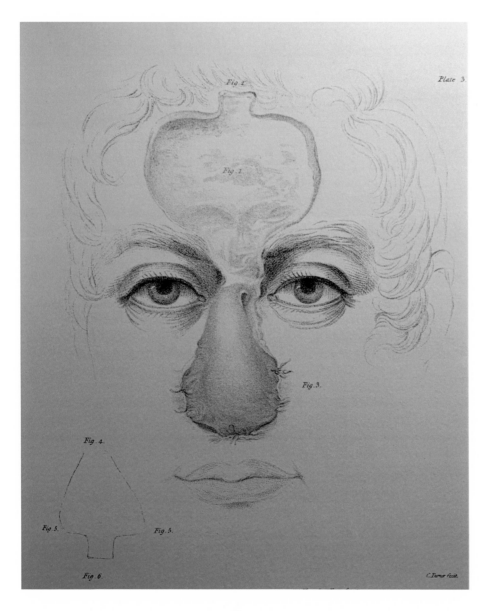

No. 30.

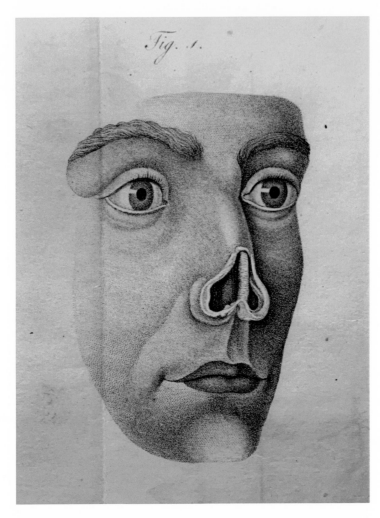

No. 31.

31. ❡ ALBERT SCHONBERG. *Sulla restituzione del naso: rapporto* [A report on the return of the nose]. Naples: Reale tipografia della Guerra, 1819.

In this early Italian book, just three years after Carpue, Schonberg recreates his early nasal reconstruction. He builds upon the work of his predecessors, Tagliacozzi, Carpue, and von Gräfe. The beautiful illustrations that accompany the book are derived from the surgery von Gräfe was performing earlier in Germany.

32. ❡ AUGUSTO FERRO. *Di autoplastica* [Autoplasty]. Rome: Tipografia Contedini, 1846.

Augusto Ferro was a prominent 19th-century Italian surgeon. In this rare book, Ferro describes his techniques in facial plastic surgery. He describes his technique for nasal reconstruction and mandible (jaw) reduction. His operations on men and women are beautifully illustrated with detailed drawings.

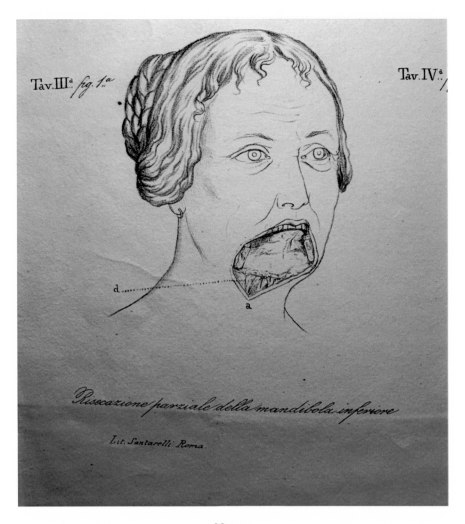

Tav. III^a fig. 1^a

Tav. IV^a

d

a

Risecazione parziale della mandibola inferiore

Lit. Santarelli Roma.

No. 32.

33. ℂ BERNHARD VON LANGENBECK. "Über eine neue Methode der totalen Rhinoplastik" [On a new Method of Total Rhinoplasty]. *Berliner klinische Wochenschrift*
1, no. 2 (January 1864).

Bernhard von Langenbeck was a 19th-century German surgeon. He specialized in ophthalmology and was also a skilled military surgeon. He succeeded Johann Dieffenbach as the director
of the Clinical Institute for Surgery and Ophthalmology at Charité in Berlin. It was at Charité
that he devised and implemented a system where recent medical graduates would reside at the
hospital as they assumed increasing responsibility in the care and supervision of surgical patients. This system led to the terms "house staff" and "residency" and earned von Langenbeck
the title "father of the surgical residency." His most famous residents were Theodor Billroth
and Emil Kocher. This house staff and residency model was adopted by William Osler and
William Halstead in the Medicine and Surgery departments at the Johns Hopkins University
Hospital later in the 19th century. In this publication, Langenbeck discusses total rhinoplasty
reconstruction addressing both the hard tissue (bony framework) and soft tissue (skin). Previous
publications addressed mostly only soft tissue reconstructions.

34. ℂ Arthur Hartmann. "Partielle Resection der Nasenscheidewand by hochgr-adiger Verkr mmung derselben" [Nasal septoplasty]. *Deutsche medizinische Wochenschrift* 8 (1882).

Arthur Hartmann was a German surgeon in the 19th century. As rhinoplasty was becoming more of a commonly performed surgical procedure, surgeons started to operate on all the other parts of the nose, including the septum, turbinates, and sinuses. Surgeons such as Gustav Killian and Otto Freer promoted this work, but it is Hartmann who is credited with first practicing the septoplasty to correct a deviated nasal septum. Prior to this surgery there were very few and ineffective means available to address this medical condition. Hartmann was also the first to perform turbinate reduction on the 1890s.

35. ℂ James Israel. "Zwei neue Methoden der Rhinoplastik" [Two new methods of rhinoplasty]. *Langenbecks Archiv für klinische Chirurgie* 53 (1896).

James Israel was a German surgeon during the latter half of the 19th and early 20th centuries. As was true of most other surgeons during this period, Israel was a military surgeon. Although a pioneer in urologic surgery, he did make significant advances in plastic surgery. In this work, Israel discusses the first free bone graft to the nose, where bone was harvested at a site away from the nose and replanted to the nose to give support for a nasal reconstruction. Without this support, a nasal reconstruction would fail because of collapse. He was also known in the field of microbiology when in 1878 he was the first to describe the disease known as actinomy-cosis in humans caused by a pathogen later named *Actinomyces israelii*.

36. ℂ Franz König. "Zur Deckung von defecten der Nasenflügel" [To cover a de-fect on the nose]. *Berliner klinische Wochenschrift* 39, no. 7 (February 1902).

Franz König was a German surgeon in the 19th century. Although mostly known for his or-thopedic surgical work involving bone and joint surgery, he did make contributions to plastic surgery. In this work, König describes the use of a composite graft, which involves the transfer of all tissue layers from one part of the body to another. Unlike a flap, where the blood supply is still attached, a graft brings no blood supply. In the nasal reconstruction performed here, a defect of the alar rim of the nose was reconstructed with a composite graft from the ear.

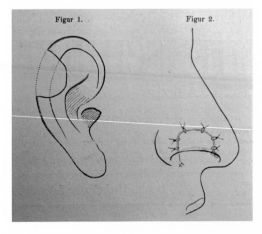

No. 36.

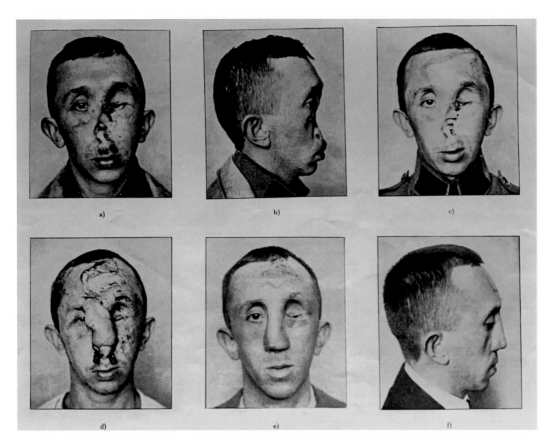

No. 37.

37. ℚ Frantıšek Burıan. *Plastická chirurgie* [Plastic surgery]. Prague: Joint Stock Printers, 1924.

František Burian was a Czech plastic surgeon in the early 20th century. In the Czech Republic, he is also known as the father of plastic surgery. Although not nearly as well known as his contemporaries, he contributed greatly to plastic surgery and ranks with Gillies, Esser, and McIndoe as one of the masters and founders of modern plastic surgery. He acquired his military surgery background during the Balkan wars of 1912–1913 and performed extensive amounts of facial reconstruction. In this work, Burian describes treatments and surgery for soldiers with extensive skull and facial injuries. His wife, Anna Lakasora-Burianova, who was among the earliest women to graduate as a doctor under the Austrian monarchy, assisted him during this period.

38. ℚ Prevot. *Quelques considerations sur la chirurgie plastique et esthetique du nez et de la face* [Some considerations on plastic and aesthetic surgery of the nose and face]. Marseille: Ed. Sergent, 1929.

Dr. Prevot was an early 20th-century French plastic surgeon who practiced at Lyon Hospital. In this small and heavily complete pamphlet, Prevot reviews the history and anatomy of facial

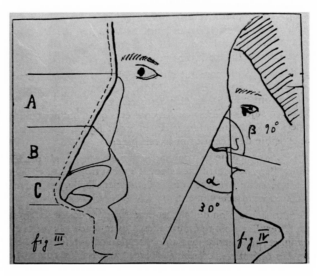

No. 38.

reconstruction. He details reconstructions of the nose, lips, and ears. Facelifts are also detailed, as is the treatment of vascular lesions of the nose. The work is complete with pre-operative and post-operative photographs, which were rarely published in France at that time.

39. ❡ JAKOB L. JOSEPH. *Nasenplastik und sonsitige Gesichitsplastik: nebst einem Anhang über Mammaplastik* [Rhinoplasty and facial plastic surgery: with an appendix on mammoplasty]. Leipzig: Curt Kabitzsch, 1931.

Jakob (or Jacques) Joseph was a German plastic surgeon in the latter part of the 19th and early 20th centuries. He was an innovator not only in plastic surgery—particularly rhinoplasty and breast surgery—but in aesthetic surgery as well. He developed the basis of cosmetic rhinoplasty as we know it today. He knew that while cosmetic surgery was not a medical necessity, it would be worth the risk to perform it if that led to a positive impact on the personality and spirit of the patient. In this extremely comprehensive work, Joseph discusses many operative techniques of both rhinoplasty and mammoplasty. The text is accompanied by numerous photographs and illustrations.

40. ❡ VICTOR FRÜHWALD. *Korrektive-kosmetische Chirurgie der Nase, Ohren und des Gesichtes* [Corrective cosmetic surgery of the nose, ears and face]. Wien: Wilhelm Maudrich, 1932.

Victor Frühwald was an Austrian plastic surgeon of the early 20th century. In this book written for surgeons wanting to learn more about facial plastic surgery, Frühwald details step-by-step instructions, with scores of illustrations, for plastic surgeons to correct deformities of the nose, ears, and face. Many different methods are discussed that had been recently discovered and improved upon. There is also a section on cosmetic surgery with descriptions on removing facial wrinkles and eyelid creases.

Cleft Lip and Palate

The history of cleft lip and palate surgery dates back to 390 BC when, for the first time, a cleft lip was closed successfully in China. Although the Egyptians and Greeks developed techniques to a remarkable degree, no descriptions of cleft operations have survived. In the Middle Ages, operations on cleft lip were described several times, and numerous descriptions of cleft lip repairs are found in European literature from the 13th to the 17th centuries, all of which fundamentally involve freshening of the cleft edges and suturing them together, with the adjunct of various dressings and salves to promote healing and combat infection. However, a successful operation on a cleft palate did not occur until 1816. This can be explained in part by the fact that cleft palates were thought to be secondary to syphilis, but also because without anesthetic, this operation was extremely painful and difficult. Gräfe and Roux published the first satisfactory result, followed by the French surgeon Veau. At the same time, other surgeons started to publish successful results by building upon the success and techniques of the others. It is because of all this past work that today's cleft lip and palate surgeries are both predictable and, more importantly, safe.

41. ⸿ PHILIBERT JOSEPH ROUX. *Mémoire sur la staphyloraphie* [Memoir of staphylorraphy]. Paris: Bechet, Migneret, 1825.

Philibert Joseph Roux was a French surgeon during the first half of the 19th century. He was trained as a military surgeon and moved to Paris, where he befriended the famous French anatomist and pathologist Xavier Bichat. In Paris he succeeded Guillaume Dupuytren as the chief surgeon at Hôtel-Dieu de Paris. Although a skilled military surgeon, he is best remembered for his work in plastic surgery, being credited for performing among the first staphylorrhaphies, the surgical repair of a cleft palate. He was also a skilled gynecologic surgeon, being credited as the first surgeon to suture a ruptured female perineum. In this work or memoir, Roux details the surgical repair of a cleft palate, where the roof of an infant's mouth remains open or patent. He improved upon the recent earlier works of cleft palate repair as performed by von Gräfe.

42. ⸿ JOHN COLLINS WARREN. "On an Operation for the Cure of Natural Fissure of Soft Palate." *American Journal of the Medical Sciences* 3, no. 5 (1828).

John Collins Warren was an American surgeon during the first half of the 19th century. He was very involved in academic medicine, being not only the founder of the *New England Journal of Medicine* but also the first dean of Harvard Medical School and the third president of the American Medical Association. Warren was also involved in two of the earlier cases of anesthesia. In 1845 he was involved in the failed use of nitrous oxide by the dentist Horace Wells. And in 1846, again at Massachusetts General Hospital, he removed a tumor from his patient's neck where Wells's competitor William Morton used ether for the first time to ease the pain from a surgical procedure. This second time, the ten-minute procedure was an anesthetic success. (Warren and Morton championed the use of sulphuric ether for surgical operations.) This work describes the first American procedure for the repair of the soft palate without any direct knowledge by Warren of Roux's description published in France three years earlier.

43. ❡ VICTOR VON BRUNS. *Chirurgischer Atlas* [Surgical atlas]. Tubingen: H. Laupp'schen, 1854.

Victor von Bruns was a German surgeon in the 19th century and a founding member of the German Society of Surgery. He is most known for his work in plastic surgery and laryngology. He gained fame with his elegant reconstructions of the lip and cheek following trauma or surgical resections for disease and cancer. He also popularized the usage of absorbent cotton dressings, which has since become normal operating practice in the treatment of wounds. In this surgical atlas, von Bruns discusses many surgeries of the head and neck. The illustrations are both exquisite and detailed.

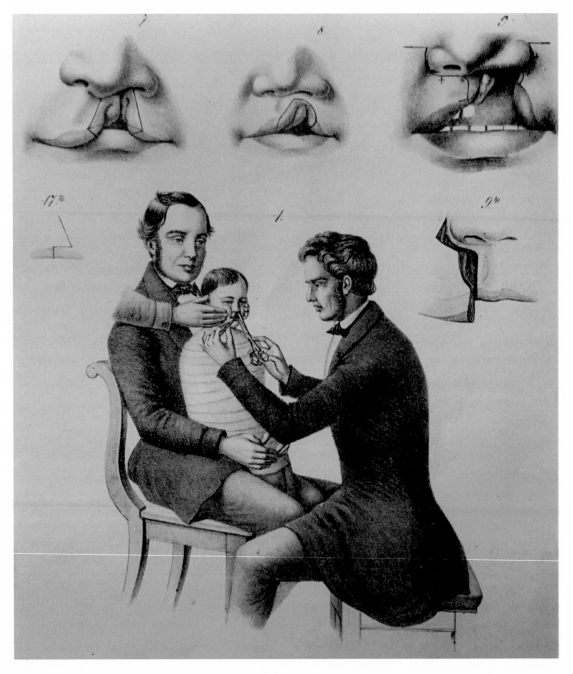

No. 43.

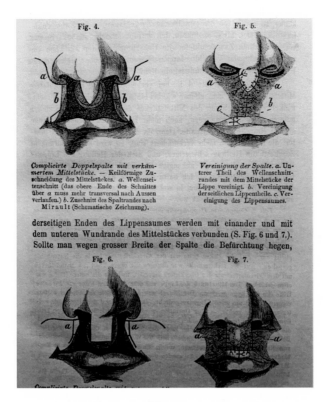

Fig. 4.

Fig. 5.

Complicirte Doppelspalte mit verkäm-
mertem Mittelstücke. — Keilförmige Zu-
schneidung des Mittelstückes. a. Wellensei-
tenschnitt (das obere Ende des Schnittes
über a muss mehr transversal nach Aussen
verlaufen.) b. Zuschnitt des Spaltrandes nach
Mirault (Schematische Zeichnung).

Vereinigung der Spalte. a. Un-
terer Theil des Wellenschnitt-
randes mit dem Mittelstücke der
Lippe vereinigt. b. Vereinigung
der seitlichen Lippentheile. c. Ver-
einigung des Lippensaumes.

derseitigen Enden des Lippensaumes werden mit einander und mit
dem unteren Wundrande des Mittelstückes verbunden (S. Fig. 6 und 7.).
Sollte man wegen grosser Breite der Spalte die Befürchtung hegen,

Fig. 6.

Fig. 7.

No. 45.

44. ❡ BERNHARD VON LANGENBECK. *Die Uranoplastik mittelst Ablösung des mucös-periostalen Gaumen berzuges* [The uranoplasty by the medial detachment of the muco-periosteum of the palate]. Berlin: August Hirschwald, 1862.

Bernhard von Langenbeck was not only known for his nasal surgery but his cleft palate surgery as well. In fact, the von Langenbeck repair still is used today for correction of the cleft palate. Cleft palate affects almost every function of the face except vision. There are different techniques based on the child's condition, but correction of the hard and soft palate remains mandatory, usually before the age of one year. In this publication, von Langenbeck describes his technique for the repair of the soft palate in the child.

45. ❡ GUSTAV SIMON. *Beitrage zur plastischen Chirurgie* [Contributions to plastic surgery]. Prague: Carl Reichenecker, 1867.

Gustav Simon was a 19th-century German surgeon. He was a military surgeon who served in reserve hospitals during the Franco-Prussian War. Simon was a well-rounded surgeon, not only performing plastic surgery but the other disciplines of orthopedics and gynecology. His military background afforded him the opportunity to publish a book informed by his early experiences on gunshot wounds. In this publication, Simon discusses his technique of preserving the cupid's bow (an important anatomic landmark of the upper lip) in the surgical repair of the cleft lip. This was the first known report detailing this preservation. Other sentinel articles appear in this publication as well.

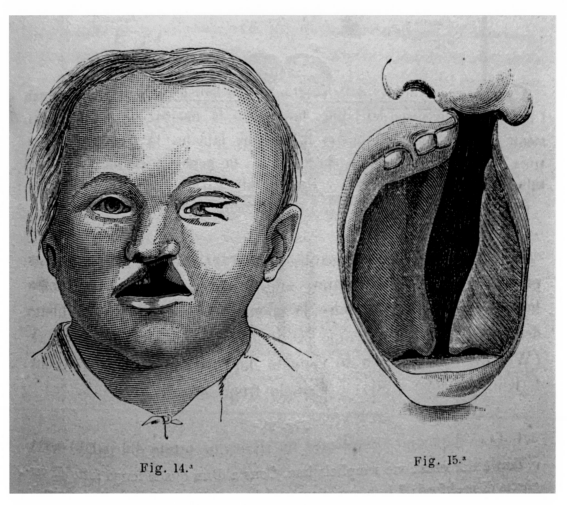

Fig. 14.ª   Fig. 15.ª

No. 46.

46. EDOARDO BASSINI. *La clinica operativa* [The operating clinic]. Genoa: Sordo-Muti, 1878.

Edoardo Bassini was an Italian surgeon during the latter half of the 19th and early 20th centuries. Like most military surgeons, he was a member of the Italian unification movement. During the war he was injured and taken prisoner. After his release and recovery, he traveled through Europe, where he studied under great European surgeons and doctors of that time including Billroth, von Langenbeck, and Lister, honing his skills. He is most well known for his description of hernia repair and is also credited for the use of eucalyptus and carbolic acid in the post-operative care of surgical patients. In this work, Bassini discusses and describes both the medical and surgical treatment of various diseases and afflictions.

47. WALTER HAGEDORN. "Über eine Modification der Hasenscharten Operation" [On a modification of the hare lip operation]. In *Tageblatt der 57. Versammlung deutscher Naturforscher und Aerzte, Magdeburg.* Leipzig: Breitkopf & Hartel, 1884.

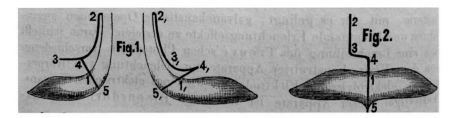

No. 47.

Werner Hagedorn was a 19th-century German surgeon. He studied in Berlin under von Langenbeck. While in Germany he was responsible for introducing the Listerian technique of antisepsis to his Magdeburg-Allstadt hospital. He was also a surgical instrument innovator, developing both the Hagedorn needle holder and the Hagedorn needle for surgery. This publication reports on Hagedorn's performing the basis for most of the early repair of a unilateral cleft lip (a cleft or hare lip on one side of the child's upper lip as opposed to the bilateral cleft lip, which involves both sides). Variations of his repair are still in use today.

48. JULES EHRMANN. Pamphlets on *palatoplastie* [palatoplasty]. Paris: Masson, 1897.

Jules Amédée Ehrmann was a French surgeon during most of the 19th century. These surgical pamphlets discuss case reports of cleft palate repair. The publications were meant for the oral surgical and plastic surgical practitioners of that time. Ehrmann published frequently on the topic of palatoplasty.

49. HAROLD GILLIES AND WILLIAM FRY. "A New Principle in the Surgical Treatment of 'Congenital Cleft Palate,' and Its Mechanical Counterpart." *British Medical Journal* 1 (1921).

Sir Harold Gillies was a 20th-century surgeon trained in otorhinolaryngology, who originally hailed from New Zealand. He has widely been regarded as the father of modern-day plastic surgery. After the start of World War I he joined the Royal Army Medical Corps and rapidly became interested in the management and repair of facial war wounds. Because of the new weaponry developed for the war and the fact that new techniques in facial reconstruction were evolving, more hospitals were needed. Gillies founded the Queen Mary's Hospital in Sidcup, London, where many techniques in both plastic surgery and facial reconstructive surgery were developed. Sir William Kelsey Fry was a 20th-century dental surgeon in World War I and a key figure in the development and advancement of oral and maxillofacial surgery. This collaboration between plastic surgeon and dental surgeon was very important in the rehabilitation of soldiers with massive facial wounds that were both destructive and disfiguring. In this work, both Gillies and Fry describe a new principle in the operation of a cleft palate. It is an important piece in that the combined expertise of both surgeons was utilized and both the maxillofacial and dental components were addressed.

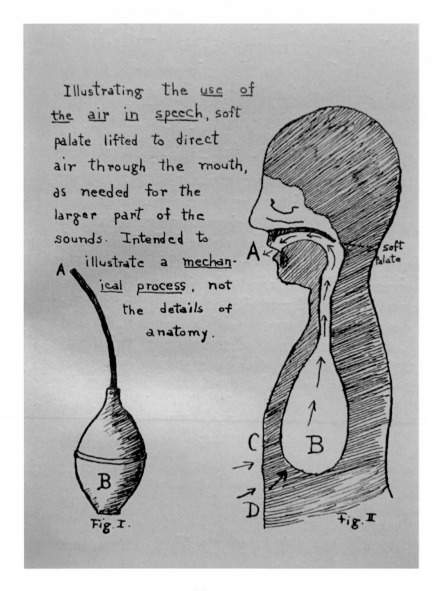

Illustrating the use of the air in speech, soft palate lifted to direct air through the mouth, as needed for the larger part of the sounds. Intended to illustrate a mechanical process, not the details of anatomy.

A

B

Fig. I.

A

soft palate

C

D

B

fig. II

No. 50.

50. ⁌ EDNA YOUNG. *Overcoming Cleft Palate Speech*. Minneapolis: Hill-Young School, 1928.

Edna Young was a 20th-century speech pathologist. She was known for her work in the moto-kinesthetic method, a version of motor speech therapy. She herself had speech problems stemming from a severe malocclusion. She had been a school teacher before transitioning to speech therapy. In this work on the correction of cleft palate speech, Young reviews the principles for overcoming speech pathology that arises particularly from a child born with a cleft palate. Children born with a cleft palate have their speech affected because of the inability to form a seal on the roof of their mouths; as such, the loss of air produces different sounds that must be overcome. Speech pathology plays a crucial role in the rehabilitation of the cleft palate patient.

51. ⁋ Victor Veau. *Division palatine* [Palatine division]. Paris: Masson, 1931.

Victor Veau was an early 20th-century French plastic surgeon. He was one of the foremost surgeons performing surgery on the cleft palate. Having performed hundreds upon hundreds of cases, he modified and improved upon the works of his predecessors, including von Langenbeck, with very high success rates. He repaired the clefts much more anatomically, leading to this high rate of success. He also believed in a collaborative approach to the success of cleft palate repair that incorporated the use of a speech pathologist in the post-operative care of his patients. In this massive volume, Veau discusses his cleft palate repair; numerous illustrations and phonetic parts written by his speech pathologist, Miss Borel, supplement the text.

52. ⁋ Arthur Le Mesurier. "A Method of Cutting and Suturing the Lip in the Treatment of Complete Unilateral Clefts." *Plastic and Reconstructive Surgery* 4 (1949).

Arthur Le Mesurier was a 20th-century pediatric surgeon who was surgical chief at the Hospital for Sick Children in Toronto, Canada. While there he worked with children born with cleft lip and palate. Previously, the restoration of the cupid's bow on a cleft repair was still challenging many surgeons. Building upon Hagedorn's method of lip repair, Le Mesurier was the first to attempt reconstruction of the cupid's bow on the vermilion of the upper lip. Before this, the repair of the cleft lip was not natural-appearing and was excessively scarred. The success of his technique was not long lived, however, as many other surgeons during the 20th century further developed surgical techniques to improve upon both the function and form of cleft lip repair.

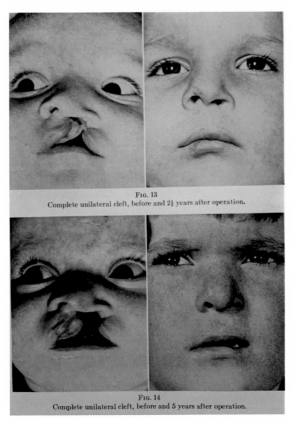

Fig. 13
Complete unilateral cleft, before and 2½ years after operation.

Fig. 14
Complete unilateral cleft, before and 5 years after operation.

No. 52.

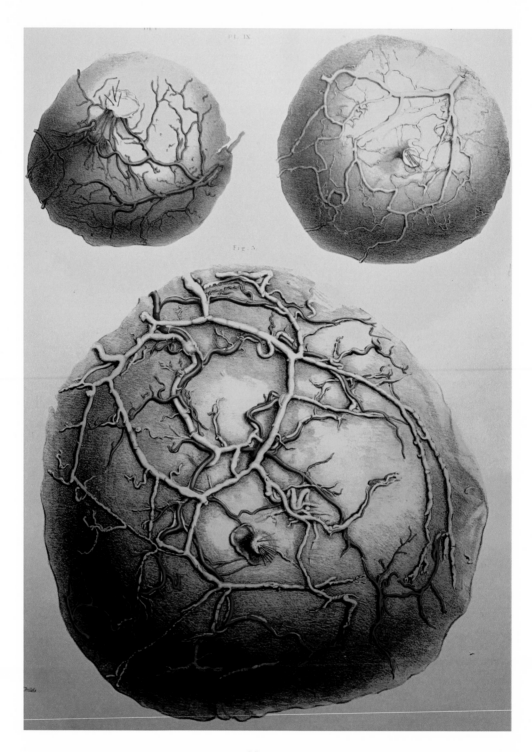

Fig. 5.

No. 54.

30

Surgery of the Breast

In 1894, William Halstead described his radical mastectomy as a treatment for breast cancer. As the understanding of breast cancer progressed, so did the interest in the reconstruction of the breast. The first attempt at a true breast reconstruction occurred in 1895. Vincent Czerny published a mastectomy case for a benign disease that was "reconstructed" by the transplantation of a fist-sized lipoma from the patient's flank. More reconstructive breast surgery followed the surgical procedure of a mastectomy or breast removal. Various flap techniques were then utilized with local and regional tissues. The early 20th century saw surgeons using the pectoral (chest wall) muscle for mound reconstruction, and abdominal wall tissue was also implemented into this approach. The only drawback for this means of reconstruction was an available supply of "donor" tissue. When breast implants were introduced in the 1960s as a means of cosmetically improving the breast, it soon became apparent that these breast implants could be used for reconstructive purposes as well.

53. ℂ JOHN PEARSON. *Practical Observations on Cancerous Complaints.* London: J. Johnson, 1793.

John Pearson was a British surgeon in the late 18th and early 19th centuries. He started his surgical apprenticeship at the age of sixteen and later on studied under John Hunter. In this book he first discusses general observations and characteristics of cancer that were known at that time. He then proceeds to discuss the ravages of cancer on various anatomic regions of the human body. Cancer of the breast, as much of it as was known at that time, is included in the discussion.

54. ℂ ASTLEY COOPER. *On the Anatomy of the Breast.* London: Longman, Orme, Green, Brown and Longmans, 1840.

Sir Astley Cooper was an early 19th-century British surgeon and anatomist. Because of these dual specialties, he was able to have a more "hands-on" approach to the teaching of anatomy rather than the previous lecture-based model. He is credited with numerous works in both those disciplines. As a student of John Hunter, he learned a great deal from him. He also took part in the formation of the Medical and Chirurgical Society of London. He was appointed surgeon to King George IV after performing surgery on him. In this anatomical textbook, Cooper writes about diseases of the breast, including exquisite, detailed illustrations. One such example is one of the earlier descriptions of hyperplastic cystic disease of the breast, which he refers to as "hydatid disease."

55. ℂ VINCENZ CZERNY. "Drei plastischen Operationen" [Three plastic surgeries]. *Verhandlungen der Deutschen Gesellschaft für Chirurgie* 24 (1895).

Vincenz Czerny was a 19th-century German Bohemian surgeon whose main contributions were in the fields of oncology and gynecologic surgery. He founded the Institut für experimentelle Krebsforschung [Institute for Experimental Cancer Research]. His work in cancer surgery is very well known, particularly after performing the first open partial nephrectomy for kidney cancer. In the field of gynecology, he was the first to perform a vaginal hysterectomy. His contributions to plastic surgery are also well known. He has been called the "Father of Plastic Surgery" for performing the first breast reconstruction. In this work, Czerny discusses the removal of a lipoma (benign fat cell tumor) and transferring it to a woman who had previously undergone a mastectomy. Czerny realized that personal appearance, not just organ reconstruction, was important in motivating a surgeon to operate upon a patient. This is a basic tenet still held and practiced today.

56. ℭ ROBERT GERSUNY. "Harte und weiche Paraffin Prothesen" (Hard and soft paraffin prostheses]. *Zentralblatt für Chirurgie* 30, no.1 (1903).

Robert Gersuny was a 19th-century German surgeon, who learned from the esteemed Theodor Billroth. He operated all over the world with Billroth and made significant contributions to both general surgery and plastic surgery. He is credited with the discovery of both paraffin and Vaseline and using them for injection into the human body. In this work he describes their use for tissue augmentation. He also describes the use of paraffin for breast augmentation, a technique that unfortunately led to disastrous results such as local reactions and tissue loss. The consequences of that procedure did great harm to the reputation of plastic surgery, which was just beginning to be recognized as a separate and distinct surgical specialty.

57. ℭ HANS KRASKE. "Die Operation der atrophischen und hypertrophischen Hängenbrust" [The operation for atrophic and hypertrophic breasts]. *Muenchener medizinische Wochenschrift*, vol. 70, no. 21 (1923).

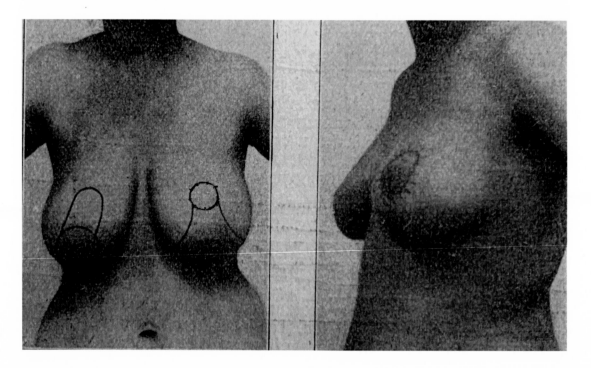

No. 57.

Hans Kraske was an early 20th-century German surgeon. His father was also a surgeon and held the Freiburg chair in surgery in the late 19th century. The younger Kraske spent many years studying both anatomy and plastic surgery. He learned under the pioneering plastic surgeon Erich Lexer. In addition to plastic surgery, Kraske was known for his orthopedic work. In this article, Kraske discusses his technique for breast reduction, the procedure to surgically reduce a large breast while also maintaining the form and function of the female breast. The areola was not touched, and the breast was sutured to the pectoralis chest muscle fascia to prevent post-operative ptosis (drooping). Up until that time, there were no safe, long-lasting procedures for breast reduction.

58. ℂ RAYMOND PASSOT. "La correction esthétique du prolapses mammaire par le procédé de la transposition du mamelon" [The aesthetic correction of a prolapsed breast by the process of transposition of the nipple]. *La presse médicale* 20 (1925).

Raymond Passot was a French plastic surgeon of the early 20th century. During this period women were becoming increasingly interested in enhancing the appearance of their breasts by reduction and lifting. Because of this trend, there was a desire to minimize the scarring on the breasts while still achieving all of the same surgical goals. In this publication, Passot discusses his procedure with a design that involves no vertical scarring. The evolution of the procedure is discussed, as are details of the surgery, including the blood supply to the breast.

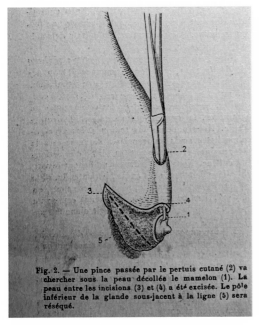

Fig. 2. — Une pince passée par le pertuis cutané (2) va chercher sous la peau décollée le mamelon (1). La peau entre les incisions (3) et (4) a été excisée. Le pôle inférieur de la glande sous-jacent à la ligne (5) sera réséqué.

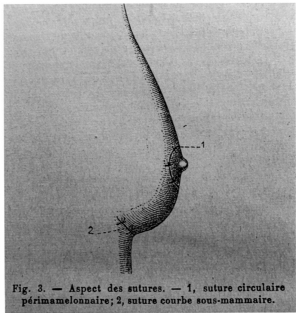

Fig. 3. — Aspect des sutures. — 1, suture circulaire périmamelonnaire; 2, suture courbe sous-mammaire.

No. 58.

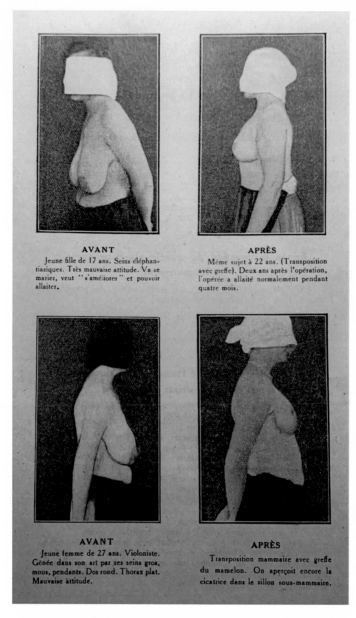

AVANT
Jeune fille de 17 ans. Seins éléphan-
tiasiques. Très mauvaise attitude. Va se
marier, veut "s'améliorer" et pouvoir
allaiter.

APRÈS
Même sujet à 22 ans. (Transposition
avec greffe). Deux ans après l'opération,
l'opérée a allaité normalement pendant
quatre mois.

AVANT
Jeune femme de 27 ans. Violoniste.
Gênée dans son art par ses seins gros,
mous, pendants. Dos rond. Thorax plat.
Mauvaise àttitude.

APRÈS
Transposition mammaire avec greffe
du mamelon. On aperçoit encore la
cicatrice dans le sillon sous-mammaire.

No. 59.

59. ❡ ANDRÉ GALAND. *La chirurgie esthétique, réparatrice et plastique du sein*
[Aesthetic breast reconstruction and aesthetic surgery]. Paris: Private health home,
1928.

André Galand was a French cosmetic surgeon in the early 20th century. In this work, Galand
describes aesthetic and reconstructive breast surgery. The techniques of breast lifting and breast
reduction are discussed. Aesthetic surgery was becoming more popular and accepted all over
the world, and it was not limited just to the face. Breast surgery was also becoming safer as
techniques involved.

60. ⁋ MAX THOREK. *Plastic Surgery of the Breast and Abdominal Wall.* Springfield, Ill.: Charles C. Thomas, 1942.

Max Thorek was a Hungarian plastic surgeon in the early 20th century and founder of the International College of Surgeons. At first an obstetrician, he later focused on general surgery and then, after World War I, his interests led him to reconstructive surgery. In this book, Thorek discusses anatomy of the chest, breast, and abdomen; he then goes on to discuss techniques related to their reconstruction following conditions caused by birth defect, illness, or disease. The publication served as a textbook meant for both student and practitioner.

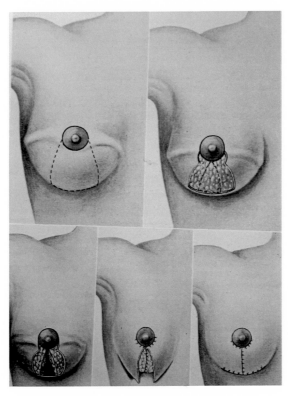

No. 60.

61. ⁋ THOMAS CRONIN AND FRANK GEROW. "Augmentation Mammaplasty: A New 'Natural Feel' Prosthesis." *Excerpta Medica International Congress* 66 (1963).

Thomas Cronin and Frank Gerow were two 20th-century American plastic surgeons. In the 1960s they collaborated with the Dow Corning Corporation to create a silicone gel breast implant product. At that time, Dow Corning specialized in silicone products. They worked to create the first breast implant that would not only augment a woman's breasts but correct for asymmetry, while also correcting for drooping to create a more uplifting profile. Surgeons began using the breast implant widely almost immediately after it reached the U.S. market in 1964, and breast augmentation quickly became one of the more popular cosmetic surgeries in the country. The creation of a silicone breast implant not only established a new branch of cosmetic surgery but also enabled women with breast cancer to undergo reconstructions to improve their

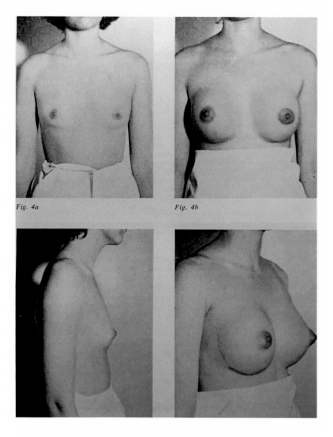

Fig. 4a   Fig. 4b

No. 61.

aesthetic appearance after cancer treatment and removal of the cancerous breast tissues. Prior to this, augmentation of the breasts had been performed with a variety of materials, often with poor results and severe health problems. This Cronin-Gerow implant had a silicone shell or envelope filled with the viscous silicone gel. In this work, which was presented at the International Society of Plastic Surgeons meeting in 1963, they discuss their initial findings on the twelve women they studied who had received the implant. There was huge interest in and acceptance of this novel procedure, and demand soon grew. Over the past fifty years, numerous changes and modifications have been made to the silicone gel breast implant, and it still remains poplar today.

62. ℭ CARL HARTRAMPF. "Breast Reconstruction with a Transverse Abdominal Island Flap." *Plastic and Reconstructive Surgery* 69 (1982).

Carl Hartrampf was a 20th-century plastic surgeon. Breast reconstruction following mastectomy had limited options. Implants were an option, but there was no predictable, long-lasting method utilizing the patient's own tissue. With the development of the TRAM (transverse rectus abdominus muscle) flap, the skin, fat, and muscle of the abdominal wall were relocated to the chest to recreate a breast mound. The tissue was transferred with its own blood supply to nourish it. The donor area from the abdomen was closed similarly to an abdominoplasty, or tummy tuck closure.

Trauma, War, and Wound Healing

Until World War I, most battle injuries were caused by small firearms or sword cuts. Facial injuries were often of little concern to survivors, who were deemed lucky enough to have escaped with their lives. Weapons utilized during World War I, such as heavy artillery and machine guns, created severe injuries on a scale never witnessed before. The circumstances of trench warfare, with men peering over parapets, caused a dramatic rise in the number of facial injuries sustained by soldiers. Shells filled with shrapnel were to blame for many of these facial and head wounds, as they were specifically designed to cause maximum damage. Hot flying metal could tear through flesh to create twisted, ragged wounds or even rip faces off entirely. Facial injuries, although very devasting, were not often as fatal as were the wounds to the chest or head. These facial injuries were not easily treated on the front line. Surgeons would sometimes stitch together a jagged wound without considering the amount of skin that had been lost, and even though the scars would heal, the skin would be contracted, pulling the face into a hideous grimace. Jaw injuries could also leave men unable to eat or drink. Some men had to be nursed sitting up to stop them from suffocating when they lay down, while others were blinded or left with a gaping hole where their nose used to be. It was because of all these wound injuries that facial reconstructive surgery and modern plastic surgery as we know it came to the forefront.

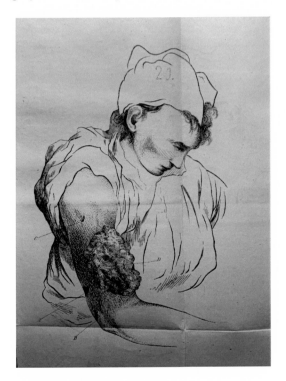

No. 63.

63. ℂ CHARLES BELL. *Gun Shot Wounds.* London: Longman, Hurst, Rees, Orme and Brown, 1814.

Sir Charles Bell, the brilliant early 19th-century Scottish surgeon and anatomist, had already made a name for himself for discovering the difference between motor (moving) nerves and sensory (feeling) nerves in the spinal cord and for describing the paralysis of the face known today as Bell's palsy. He was also a gifted artist. In this book we have a rare example of both a practicing surgeon and an artist depicting the effects and toll of war on the human body. The paintings are stark and haunting; they serve as a reminder of what these open battles were like and the destruction rendered. Because of such war wounds during and after World War I, modern plastic surgery made many of its greatest advances.

64. ℭ CLAUDE LALLEMAND. *Plaie à la face avec perte de substance* [Plague on the face with loss of substance]. Paris: Bechet, Migneret, 1824.

Claude Lallemand was an early 19th-century French surgeon who served in the armies of the Empire. He also trained under the famous French surgeon Guillaume Dupuytren. In this work, Lallemand describes in great detail a facial reconstruction of a young female, who had lost part of her cheek and lower lip from a spreading, malignant pustule.

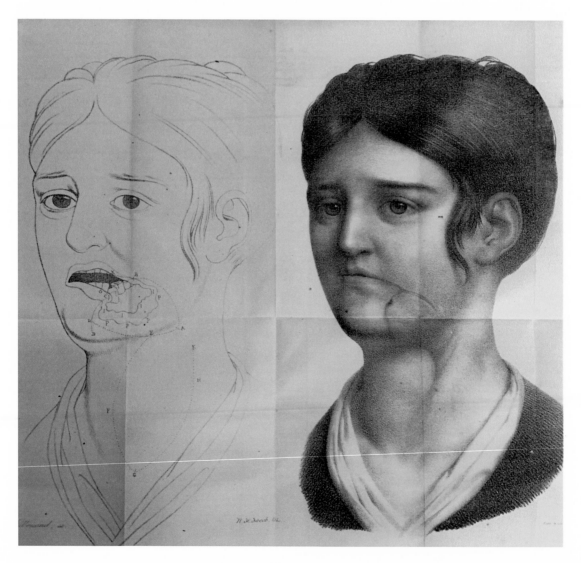

No. 64.

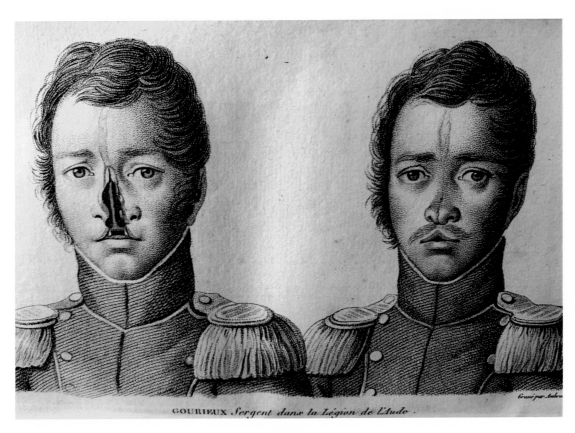

GOURIEUX *Sergent dans la Légion de l'Aude.*

Gravé par Ambro.

No. 65.

65. ℭ DOMINIQUE LARREY. *Clinique chirurgicale* [Surgical clinic]. Vol. 2. Paris: Chez Gabon, 1830.

Baron Dominique Jean Larrey was a 19th-century French military surgeon. He served in Napoleon's Grande Armée and was an important innovator in battlefield medicine and triage. He has often been considered the first modern military surgeon. Larrey initiated modern methods of army surgery, field hospitals, and army ambulance corps. He formulated the rules for triage of war casualties, treating the wounded according to the immediate urgency of need for medical care regardless of rank or nationality. This method of triage is still in use today. Larrey's writings are still regarded as valuable sources of surgical and medical knowledge and have been translated into many modern languages. Between 1800 and 1840, he published at least twenty-eight books or articles. His son Hippolyte was surgeon-in-ordinary to the emperor Napoleon III. In this volume Larrey discusses his manner of performing a nasal reconstruction. Instrumentation used for the surgery is also discussed.

66. ℭ CHARLES DELALAIN. *Perte du nez et des yeux* [Loss of nose and eyes]; *Prothese de la bouche et de la face* [Prosthesis of the mouth and face]. Paris: Philipona, 1882.

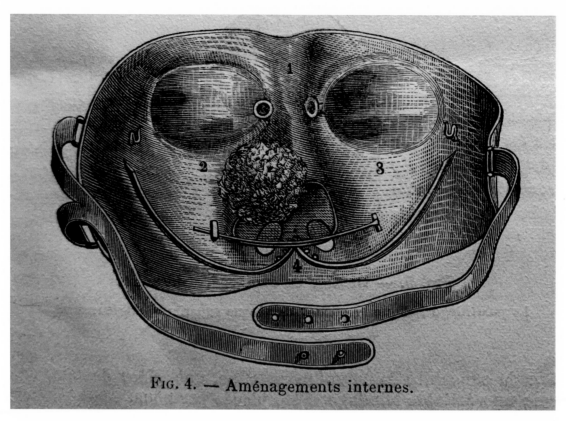

FIG. 4. — Aménagements internes.

No. 66.

Charles Delalain was a French surgeon-dentist in the late 19th century. This work, extracted from the review in *L'odontologie*, is extremely rare. The mask was made in silver and the eyes made of glass. The denture for the teeth was made of vulcanite. The mask sought to replace the areas of the face that were lost or injured from accidents of war. This book also details the description of how to apply the mask.

67. ℂ FELIX MARCHAND. *Der Process der Wundheilung* [The process of wound healing]. Stuttgart: Verlag von Ferdinand Enke, 1901.

Felix Marchand was a German pathologist of the late 19th and early 20th centuries. He rose to prominence at the pathological institutes in both Halle and Leipzig. He is best known for coining the term *atherosclerosis*—from the Greek *athero* (meaning gruel) and *sclerosis* (meaning hardening)—to describe the fatty substance leading to hardening and narrowing of the arteries. In this pathologic textbook, Marchand describes wound healing from the vantage point of a pathologist. He discusses the origin and progression of wound healing from what was known at that time. Surgeons and doctors for years had been discussing wound healing, and it continues to play a significant role in the practice of every plastic surgeon today.

68. ℂ LÉON DUFOURMENTEL. *Chirurgie d'urgence des blessures de la face et du cou* [Emergency surgery for face and neck injuries]. Paris: A. Maloine et fils, 1918.

Léon Dufourmentel was a 20th-century French surgeon who specialized in maxillofacial surgery and reconstructive surgery. He trained at the hospitals of Paris and then led the clinical faculty of medicine in Paris. During World War I, he was responsible for caring for the *gueules cassées* (broken faces), which led to the creation of units of maxillofacial surgery. He is also responsible for utilizing a method for the repair of facial wounds. In this method, he described a pedicled vascularized flap from the temporal scalp (popularly called a Dufourmentel flap) and transferred the tissue to the chin area. This tissue transfer was more reliable than a free skin graft. It was his idea to first use prosthetic devices where reconstructions with autogenous tissue failed. The implants used were mostly made of ivory and rubber. In this book, Dufourmentel shares the care and reconstructions performed on those injured.

69. ℂ Harold Gillies. *Plastic Surgery of the Face.* London: Frowde, Hodder and Stoughton, 1920.

Considered by many to be the father of modern plastic surgery, Sir Harold Gillies wrote this epic book for surgeons wishing to specialize in plastic surgery. In the early 20th century, plastic surgery was in its infancy and practiced by general surgeons. The advent of World War I brought with it more facial and head injuries than previously because soldiers were in trenches with their heads exposed to new and more powerful weapons. In 1916, Britain officially recognized

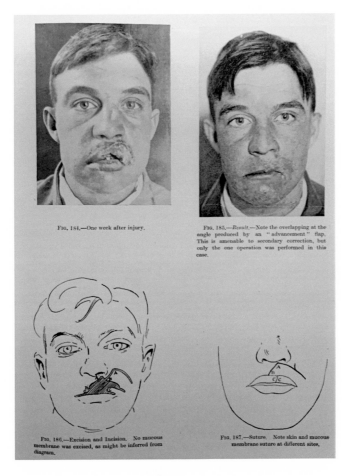

Fig. 184.—One week after injury.

Fig. 185.—*Result.*—Note the overlapping at the angle produced by an "advancement" flap. This is amenable to secondary correction, but only the one operation was performed in this case.

Fig. 186.—Excision and Incision. No mucous membrane was excised, as might be inferred from diagram.

Fig. 187.—Suture. Note skin and mucous membrane suture at different sites.

No. 69.

plastic surgery as a specialty with the founding of the military hospital in Aldershot. Gillies was an ear, nose, and throat specialist from New Zealand who was at the forefront of this new-found specialty. Gillies treated thousands of patients during his time at Aldershot. In this book, he records those experiences, his goal being to share the skills and techniques learned and mastered there. Each anatomic area of the face is depicted with case studies and photographs. Gillies employed skin grafts, flap transfers, tubed surgeries, and even facial prostheses. The advent of antisepsis and anesthesia made these surgeries possible.

70. ℭ HENRY PICKERALL. *Facial Surgery.* New York: William Wood and Co., 1924.

Henry Pickerall was a 20th-century plastic surgeon also from New Zealand. Although not as well known as the other "fathers" of plastic surgery, such as Gillies, McIndoe and Kilner, Pickerall did advance the specialty of facial reconstructive surgery. He was, in fact, the first maxillofacial surgeon in New Zealand. Like Gillies's, this book was meant to discuss and detail the diagnosis, care, and surgical management of the face. He drew upon his vast experience treating those injured during the war.

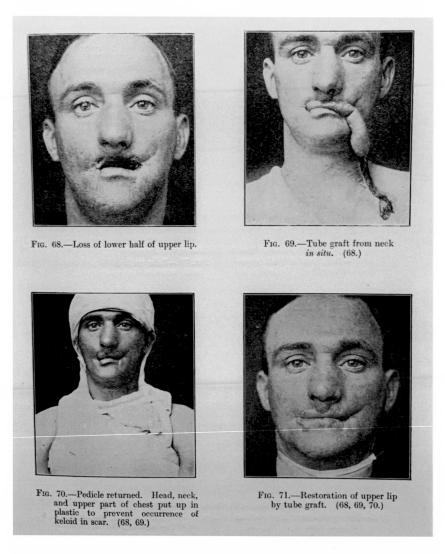

FIG. 68.—Loss of lower half of upper lip.

FIG. 69.—Tube graft from neck *in situ.* (68.)

FIG. 70.—Pedicle returned. Head, neck, and upper part of chest put up in plastic to prevent occurrence of keloid in scar. (68, 69.)

FIG. 71.—Restoration of upper lip by tube graft. (68, 69, 70.)

No. 70.

71. ℭ VILRAY BLAIR. "Use and Uses of Large Split-skin Grafts of Intermediate Thickness." *Surgery, Gynecology & Obstetrics* 49 (1929).

Vilray Blair was a 20th-century American plastic surgeon specializing in head, face, and oral reconstruction. He was one of the pioneers of modern plastic surgery; his training was occurring during the time of rapid advancements in the specialty. He is credited with many oral and maxillofacial procedures, but in this publication Blair specifically advances the technique of skin grafting. It had been over eighty years since Reverdin used his "pinch grafts," and since then the techniques had advanced. Blair now advocates thicker split thickness skin grafts. Because of this increased thickness, the applicability of the graft increased. General surgeons were using grafts as well, and the invention of the dermatome helped to create an even thickness of skin that measured approximately fifteen-thousandths of an inch. Burn surgery and rehabilitation was greatly facilitated with the use of skin grafts.

72. ℭ JOHANNES ESSER. *Biologic or Artery Flaps of the Face.* Monaco: Institut Esser de chirurgie structive, 1935.

Johannes "Jan" Esser was a 20th-century Dutch plastic surgeon who was credited with many innovative methods of reconstructive surgery on soldiers wounded in World War I. He was a true Renaissance man by being not only a skilled plastic surgeon but also a chess champion and art dealer. He practiced all over the world before settling in Germany. His reconstructive surgical techniques are still employed today, especially with the use of the flap, which is a piece of tissue still attached to its blood supply and transferred to another area of the body in need of that tissue. In this beautifully illustrated and bound book and atlas, Esser describes scores of cases using these flaps for their reconstruction. This book was intended for the new practitioners to reconstructive facial plastic surgery.

73. ℭ MACHTELF SANO. "Skin Grafting, a New Method Based on the Principles of Tissue Culture." *American Journal of Surgery* 61 (1943).

Machteld Sano was a 20th-century Belgian physician who sought to advance the principles of skin grafting with the introduction of a fibrin glue that would remove the previous requirement of sutures and pressure dressing for the success of skin grafts. Prior to this, skin grafting was technically very challenging. Here we have the improvement of a surgical technique by use of a biologic substance rather than surgical advancement.

Cosmetic Surgery and Facial Rejuvenation

The early twentieth century saw a demand for cosmetic surgery, especially facial rejuvenation. During this time, facelifts were performed by simply pulling on the skin on the face and cutting the loose parts off. The first facelift was reportedly performed by Eugen Holländer in 1901. An elderly Polish female aristocrat asked him to "lift her cheeks and corners of the mouth." After much debate, he finally proceeded to excise an elliptical piece of skin around the ears. It was crude, but effective. Facelifts were often done in secrecy because both the patient and surgeon did not want to publicize the fact. Eventually, in 1907, a textbook totally devoted to facial cosmetic surgery was published by Charles Miller. In 1919, a more formal facelift procedure was described by Raymond Passot. This led to many others writing about their version of the technique. The first female plastic surgeon, Suzanne Noël, also played a large role in the development of facial cosmetic surgery.

74. ℂ DAVID PRINCE. *Plastics: A New Classification and a Brief Exposition of Plastic Surgery.* Philadelphia: Lindsay and Blakiston, 1868.

David Prince was an American military surgeon who served under General McClellan during the Civil War. Prince, who was very progressive in his ideas, was a strong proponent of antisepsis and the use of ether. His Prince Infirmary treated over three thousand patients a year, and he consequently had considerable experience in burn surgery and cleft palate surgery. In this book, Prince discusses various topics in plastic surgery, with a heavy emphasis and detailed discussions of rhinoplasty and cheiloplasty (lip surgery). Other topics in plastic surgery are reviewed as well.

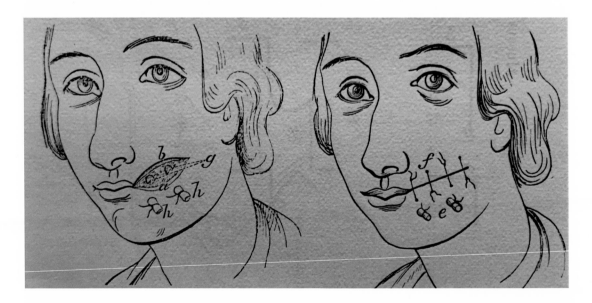

No. 74.

75. ℭ CHARLES DARWIN. *The Expression of the Emotions in Man and Animals.* London: John Murray, 1872.

Charles Robert Darwin was an English geologist, naturalist, and biologist who is best known for his contributions to the science of evolution. His groundbreaking book, *On the Origin of Species,* was published in 1859. In *The Expression of Emotions,* which was his third work on evolutionary theory, Darwin studies the biologic aspects of emotional life, including such mannerisms as raising an eyebrow in surprise or blushing when embarrassed. These physical findings may be sought after when a surgeon performs surgery on the face to recreate a certain characteristic or trait, and this book is the first to discuss the biology behind it.

76. ℭ THOMAS SOZINSKEY. *Personal Appearance and the Culture of Beauty.* Philadelphia: Allen, Lane and Scott, 1877.

Thomas Sozinskey was a late 19th-century physician and author. In this book meant for the layperson, Sozinsky describes what makes each part of the human body beautiful. He has chapters dedicated to men and women individually and then not only discusses each part of the face but also writes about the teeth and skin. His is a purely subjective analysis, but this is important since at that time more physicians and surgeons were starting to deal with the art of cosmetic and aesthetic surgery. He discusses human beauty as it was presented to us through ages past by painters, sculptors, and artists.

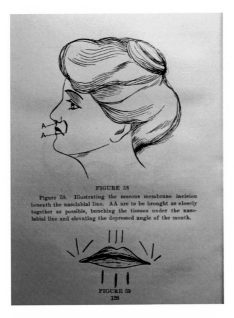

No. 77.

77. ℭ CHARLES MILLER. *The Correction of Featural Imperfections.* Chicago: Charles Miller (Oak Printing Co.), 1907.

Charles Miller was an early 20th-century plastic surgeon credited with the first textbook specifically related to cosmetic surgery. The work was ahead of its time, and it was criticized for discussing procedures that were not life preserving or altering. The specialty was even considered "quackery" by many of the other general and reconstructive surgeons of that time. Many others in the medical community also considered Miller a quack, putting him in a similar category as Woodward and Crum even though he had formal training and his procedures were sound. In this book, Miller addresses the correction and rejuvenation of the eyes, ears, cheek, face, and neck, with procedures on both the skin and muscle.

78. ℭ JOHN WOODBURY. *Beauty Culture*. New York: G. W. Dillingham Co., 1910.

John H. Woodbury was an American self-trained dermatologist in the late 19th and early 20th centuries. In his youth he had a large facial nevus, or mole, on his face. His self-esteem improved after successfully having it removed, and he realized the significance that surgery can have on a person's life. He built an empire of cosmetic surgery institutes in six states, with scores of physicians and employees. He and his colleagues performed numerous facial cosmetic surgeries of the face, forehead, cheek, nose, and chin. These procedures were described not in peer-reviewed journals and books but rather through advertisements for the public, and so he was fairly unknown in medical and academic circles. In addition, he started a proprietary cosmetic line that was very lucrative and was later sold to the Jergens Company. In this book, Woodbury discusses both dermatologic and surgical means to restore and maintain facial rejuvenation. Not only does he discuss topical creams, ointments, and medications, but he also discusses electrolysis, vibrations, and message. He also considers surgery, but not with the reverence that other true surgeons of the day were practicing. He incorporated all these modalities into his practices, so it is easy to see why he maintained a large following. Eventually this type of practicing and advertising became illegal, and his practices started to fail; he later admitted he was not even a medical doctor. Despite this infamy, he did have historically significant achievements.

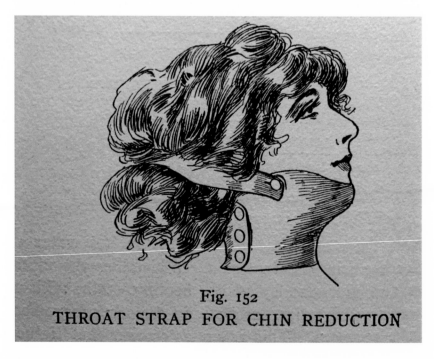

Fig. 152
THROAT STRAP FOR CHIN REDUCTION

No. 78.

79. ℂ Frederick Kolle. *Plastic and Cosmetic Surgery.* New York: Appleton and Co., 1911.

Frederick Kolle was a late 19th-/early 20th-century German plastic surgeon who initially had radiology training and was one of the first pioneers of x-ray technology. Kolle maintained an active practice in plastic surgery, and his impetus for writing this book was his feeling that there ought to be an authoritative textbook on the art of plastic surgery, which was quickly becoming more and more popular. He helped to legitimize plastic surgery as a specialty, and his writing a formal textbook describing detailed accounts and methods of plastic surgery would aid in this endeavor. He references surgical procedures from the preceding hundreds of years. In his attempt to publish an authoritative book, Kolle not only describes plastic surgical procedures but also discusses requirements for operating in the operating room and lays out principles of antisepsis, anesthetics, dressings, instrumentation and post-operative care.

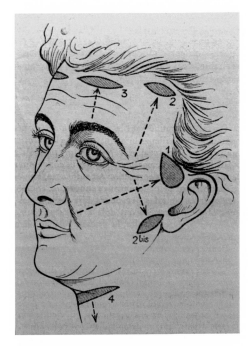

No. 80.

80. ℂ Raymond Passot. "La chirurgie esthétique des rides du visage" [Aesthetic surgery of facial wrinkles]. *La presse médicale* 27 (1919).

Raymond Passot was an early 20th-century French plastic surgeon. Along with Dr. Hippolyte Morestin, Passot was responsible for advancing the field of plastic surgery in France. In the early 20th century, cosmetic surgery was becoming increasingly popular, as was facial rejuvenation. This led to surgeons with large egos debating who performed the first facelift. Hollander claimed to have performed a facelift in 1901 on a Polish aristocrat, and Lexer claimed to have performed one in 1906 for an actress. Even the esteemed Joseph claimed one in 1912. But despite those claims, in 1919 Passot first published this article, appearing in *La presse médicale*, which describes the details in full. This procedure details where the incisions were made, then goes on to discuss the elevation and redraping of the skin. Today's facelifts may be more advanced and sophisticated—and safer—yet the objectives remain the same.

81. ℂ CHARLES WILLI. *Facial Rejuvenation.* Somerset: Purnell and Sons, 1926.

Charles Willi was another surgeon of question in the early 20th century despite publishing books on plastic surgery and even maintaining a successful plastic surgery practice for over fifty years. His claim to have earned a medical degree in the United States was later deemed false because the head of the awarding university was convicted of running a fake diploma mill and thus Willi's qualification was bogus. This led to a prosecution and fine but, because of a loophole in British law, Willi was able to practice plastic surgery as long as he did not willfully pass himself off as a physician or surgeon. In this book on facial rejuvenation Willi, however one regards his training and background, does discuss in detail many facial plastic surgery operations complete with pre-operative and post-operative photographs. Willi and these other so-called "beauty docs" did practice with the advantage of allowing them to advertise where other physicians could not. The one major disadvantage was an inability to work with anesthetists and use general anesthesia, so these facial cosmetic procedures were performed under local anesthesia only. Anesthesiologists risked loss of license if known to practice with these unlicensed doctors. Even with the limitation of local anesthesia only, Willi was also known to have performed some "breast firming" procedures.

82. ℂ JOSIF GINSBURG. *The Hygiene of Youth and Beauty.* Sydney, Australia: Cornstalk Publishing Co., 1927.

Josif Ginsburg was an early 20th-century Russian trauma and military surgeon who later turned his talents and skills to the rapidly growing field of cosmetic surgery. He relocated his practice to Los Angeles in the 1920s and, with the advent of Hollywood and movie stars demanding more cosmetic surgery, his practice thrived. In this book, like the other books involving cosmetic surgery, the emphasis is more on the non-academic and non-medical aspects of the field of plas-

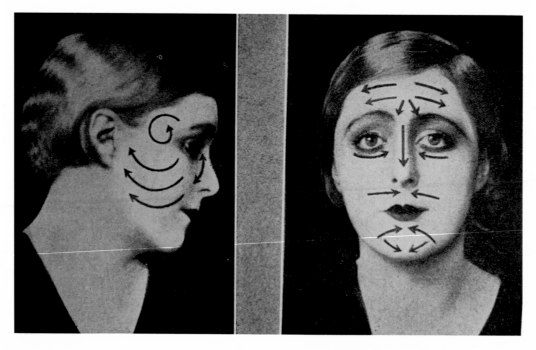

No. 82.

tic surgery. The writing addresses both surgical and non-surgical methods for restoring and rejuvenating not only the skin but facial complexion and hair as well. Chemical peels and skin care are also discussed.

83. ℭ CHARLES MILLER. *Doctor Charles Conrad Miller's Review of Plastic and Esthetic Surgery.* Philadelphia: F. A. Davis and Co., 1927.

Charles Miller was also an eager publicist. In the inaugural issue of this softbound journal, he not only discusses cosmetic surgical procedures but also general surgical procedures for the practitioner. His journal is filled with medical and non-medical advertisements as well.

84. ℭ J. HOWARD CRUM. *The Making of a Beautiful Face.* New York: Walton Book Co., 1928.

J. Howard Crum was another of the so-called Beauty Docs of the early 20th century. He was a huge fan of publicity and would publicize the surgeries he performed. Like other practitioners of the time, he was frowned upon by the more legitimate practitioners; yet he did command a solid following. In this book, Crum discusses the medical, dermatologic, and surgical factors that go into making a beautiful face.

85. ℭ RAYMOND PASSOT. *Chirurgie esthétique pure* [Pure aesthetic surgery]. Paris: Chez Gaston Doin, 1931.

In this book Raymond Passot again reveals his expertise for cosmetic surgery. Not only are surgical techniques discussed, but Passot also shares with the reader how he examines patients and reveals his suturing techniques. Passot was very proud of his results, as is evidenced by actual before-and-after pictures of patients undergoing both facial cosmetic surgery and breast cosmetic surgery. At that time, breast enhancement procedures were limited to the correction of sagging breasts or enlarged breasts. It would be another thirty years until breast augmentation with implants would be performed.

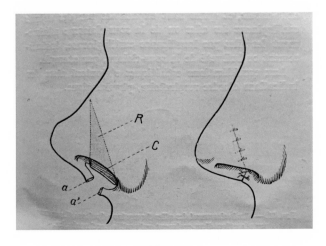

NO. 85.

49

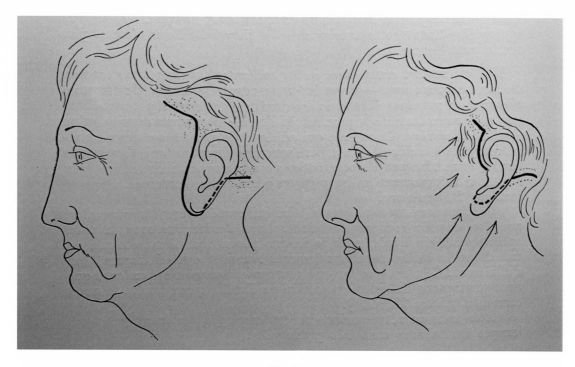

NO. 86.

86. ℭ JULIEN BOURGUET. *La véritable chirurgie esthétique du visage* [The real aesthetic facial surgery]. Paris: Les petits-fils de Plon et Nourrit, 1936.

Julien Bourguet was a French surgeon in the 20th century. In this book Bourguet discusses cosmetic surgery of the nose, ears, eyes, mandible (chin), and face. Bourguet performed a lot of aesthetic surgery in France. Both the hard and soft tissues of the face are addressed. As medical photography was becoming more standard, the book is filled with numerous before-and-after pictures. This technique of "before-and-after" pictures has become the standard in today's cosmetic surgery practices.

87. ℭ HENRY SCHIRESON. *Your New Face Is Your Fortune*. Philadelphia: Franklin House, 1947.

Henry Schireson was also an early 20th-century "Beauty Doc." Like Willi, he had little formal training and practiced outside professional organized medicine. He did not belong to professional societies and maintained no hospital privileges. He did not author articles or teach at medical schools. He was simply a flamboyant personality who advertised greatly and performed cosmetic surgery. Schireson rose to fame in 1923 when he operated on the nose of vaudeville star Fanny Brice. Alas, he too ran afoul of the law. He had legal trouble with his license and faced mounting malpractice claims. In this manual, he discusses the virtues of having a more perfect nose.

Anesthesia, Instrumentation, and Nursing

Every surgeon knows he is a member of a team. More than anything, a successful surgical result is achieved when there is a concerted effort. The team in the operating room consists of surgeons, anesthesiologists, and a skilled and dedicated group of nurses and assistants. Advancements in anesthesia during the 1800s, even with all its controversy, helped to pave the way for the progress made in plastic surgery today, which was in turn made possible by the unwavering help and support of nurses and medical professionals. Instrumentation and technology also evolved and played a large role in the implementation of surgical procedures. The surgeons of the 16th century may not immediately recognize the operating rooms of today, but they would certainly appreciate them.

88. ℂ MARTIN GAY. *A Statement of the Claims of Charles T. Jackson, M.D., to the Discovery of the Applicability of Sulphuric Ether to the Prevention of Pain in Surgical Operations.* Boston: David Clapp, 1847.

Martin Gay was a 19th-century physician with a background in chemistry and mineralogy. The truth mattered very much to Gay, and he felt the need to opine on the great ether controversy that was swirling around the surgical and medical world in the mid-19th century. He wanted to defend Charles Jackson and his discovery of sulfuric ether. Two men claimed to have discovered ether and etherization for anesthesia: Jackson and William T. G. Morton. Gay defends Jackson as the person who invented it in this thesis.

89. ℂ JOSEPH AND HENRY LORD. *A Defense of Jackson's Claims to the Discovery of Etherization.* Boston: Littell's Living Age, 1848.

Joseph Lord and Henry Lord were noted 19th-century Boston attorneys who penned this treatise giving support to Charles Jackson as the true discoverer of ether. There was a great debate over who deserved the credit for discovering ether anesthesia. Joseph and Henry Lord's defense of Jackson's claim was first published as an article in the periodical *Littell's Living Age* under the title "The Ether Discovery." This separate edition contains an appendix that was not included in the periodical version. The two Lords collected testimony showing that Jackson, rather than his rival Warren T. G. Morton, was the true discoverer of ether anesthesia.

90. ℂ JOHN COLLINS WARREN. *Etherization.* Boston: William D. Ticknor and Co., 1848.

John Collins Warren was a 19th-century American surgeon and founder of the *New England Journal of Medicine.* He was the third president of the American Medical Association and the first dean of Harvard Medical School. Warren was involved not once but twice in the earliest history of anesthesia. The first incident was a failed demonstration of nitrous oxide by dentist Horace Wells on January 20, 1845. Not willing to accept that failure, on October 16,

1846, Warren agreed to perform a public demonstration of a surgical operation again on a patient using anesthesia, this time under ether anesthesia administered by Wells's colleague and competitor, William T. G. Morton. The operation lasted about ten minutes and the patient was seemingly unconscious for its duration. Warren's personal journal for this day records, "Did an interesting operation at the Hospital this morning, while the patient was under the influence of Dr. Morton's preparation to prevent pain. The substance employed was sulphuric ether." Warren was quick to see the remarkable advantages offered by ether in surgical procedures, and he then championed the cause of etherization through this work and other publications.

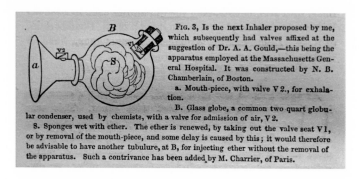

FIG. 3, Is the next Inhaler proposed by me, which subsequently had valves affixed at the suggestion of Dr. A. A. Gould,—this being the apparatus employed at the Massachusetts General Hospital. It was constructed by N. B. Chamberlain, of Boston.

a. Mouth-piece, with valve V 2., for exhalation.

B. Glass globe, a common two-quart globular condenser, used by chemists, with a valve for admission of air, V 2.

S. Sponges wet with ether. The ether is renewed, by taking out the valve seat V 1, or by removal of the mouth-piece, and some delay is caused by this; it would therefore be advisable to have another tubulure, at B, for injecting ether without the removal of the apparatus. Such a contrivance has been added by M. Charrier, of Paris.

NO. 91.

91. ℂ CHARLES JACKSON. *A Manual of Etherization*. Boston: J. B. Mansfield, 1861.

Charles Jackson was not only a noted physician but an active geologist and chemist. He had first used sulfuric ether on himself following an accidental inhalation of chlorine gas. He realized that insensibility could be achieved and be useful for anesthesia. Unfortunately, William T. G. Morton also laid claim to its discovery, and Jackson spent most of the remainder of his life attempting to earn that credit. In this manual, Jackson writes with a view to both the surgeon and the soldier about the effects of anesthetic agents.

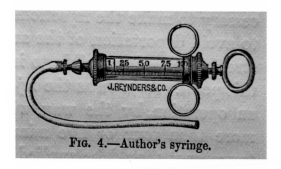

FIG. 4.—Author's syringe.

NO. 92.

92. ℂ JAMES CORNING. *Local Anesthesia in General Medicine and Surgery*. New York: Appleton and Co., 1886.

James Corning was an American neurologist known mainly for his early experiments on neuraxial blockade. When the American Civil War began in 1861, Corning's family moved to Stuttgart, Germany. Corning experimented with regional anesthesia. Like the ether controversy that was swirling around in the mid-19th century, so, too, was there controversy about who was the first to describe local anesthesia. In 1884 Karl Koller described the anesthetic properties of cocaine. In 1898 August Bier performed surgery under spinal anesthesia. Following the publication of Bier's experiments, a controversy developed about whether Corning or Bier had performed the first successful spinal anesthetic. In this book, Corning avoids the controversy as he discusses local anesthesia and pain.

93. ℂ ERNST BLASIUS. *Akiurgische Abbildungen, oder, Darstellung der blutigen chirurgischen Operationen . . .* [Surgical illustrations, or, Representation of bloody surgical operations]. Berlin: Verlag von Friedrich August Herbig, 1833.

Ernst Carl Friedrich Blasius was a 19th-century German surgeon. After several years of military medical service, he relocated to the University of Halle, where he rose to the rank of full professor. He made numerous contributions to surgery. In this atlas, he generously depicts and illustrates surgical instruments and discusses surgical technology and technique with a heavy emphasis on plastic and reconstructive surgery.

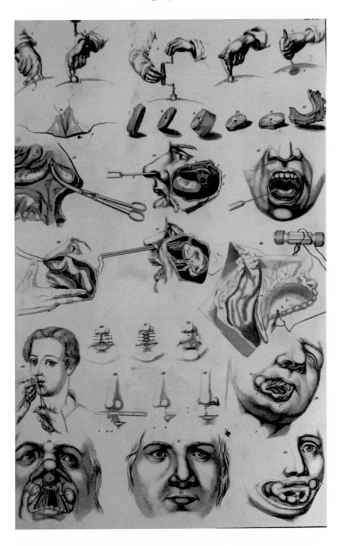

No. 93.

94. ℂ James Sims. *Silver Sutures in Surgery.* New York: Samuel S. and William Wood, 1858.

James Marion Sims was a 19th-century American surgeon, known as the father of modern gynecology. He developed a surgical treatment for vesico-vaginal fistulas in the early 19th century. These fistulas were a relatively common condition, in which a woman's urine leaked into her vaginal cavity from her bladder; in the 1800s, many regarded the fistulas as untreatable. After years of effort to repair the fistulas with different techniques and procedures, Sims developed an improved surgical operation. He also popularized the use of silver metal sutures to treat and cure women who had these vesico-vaginal fistulas. Sims's surgical cure for vesico-vaginal fistulas eased both the social stigma and physical discomfort of many affected women. Current treatments of vesico-vaginal fistulas have evolved since the 19th century, yet some of the basic principles utilized by Sims have been incorporated into today's surgeries.

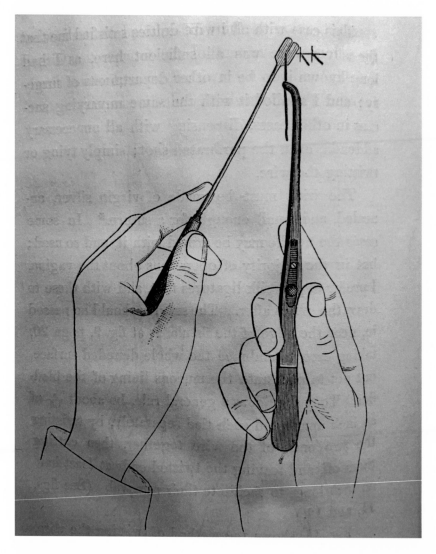

No. 94.

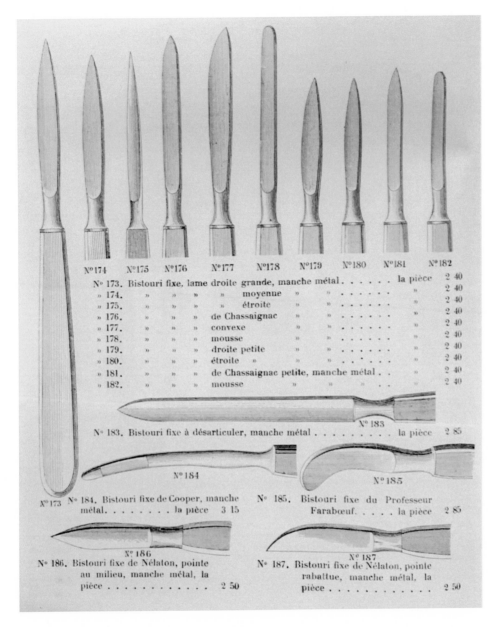

No. 95.

95. ❡ GEMBLOUX. *Catalogue général illustré d'instruments de chirurgie* [General illustrated catalogue of surgical instruments]. Paris: Auguste Legros, 1905.

Gembloux is a municipality in Belgium. Around 1875, Louis-Joseph Mathieu had established a workshop in Paris for the manufacture of surgical instruments that quickly expanded. Around 1880, he returned to Namur to hire a worker and was unsuccessful. He then went to Gembloux and hired Dieudonné Simal. They began to be known for their surgical instruments for the eyes, nose, throat, and ears. Simal later hired his brother-in-law, Guibert Legros, and Legros's brother, Auguste, to come and work with them. This catalogue details and illustrates some of the great instruments manufactured in Gembloux for use in plastic surgery.

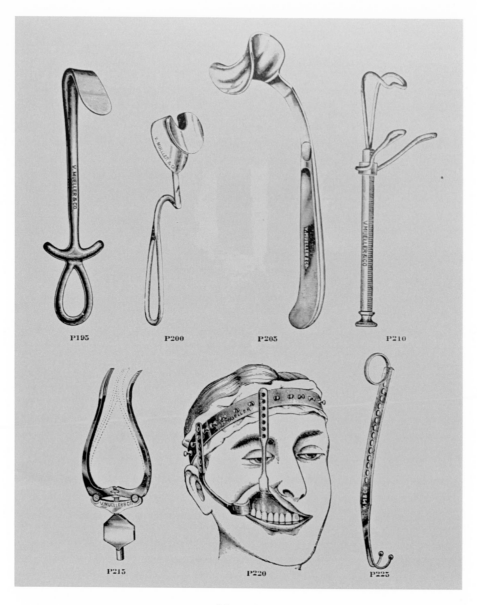

No. 96.

96. ℂ MUELLER. *Instruments for Oral and Plastic Surgery.* Chicago: Mueller and Co., 1928.

In 1893, Vinzenz Mueller brought his knowledge of German instrument craftsmanship to the United States and established a tradition that has carried through to today. His successor, William Merz, established the V. Mueller name as one synonymous with innovation and collaboration. In 1951, Leonard Snowden and George Pencer introduced the revolutionary tungsten carbide insert to the jaws of surgical instruments to make them stronger and longer lasting. Over the decades surgical instruments have become more sophisticated and more advanced. Despite so many innovations, there are still instruments today that have barely evolved. This catalogue shows instruments for the practitioners of plastic surgery and oral surgery, including maxillofacial surgery.

97. ℂ FLORENCE NIGHTINGALE. *Notes on Nursing*. Boston: William Carter, 1860.

Florence Nightingale is recognized as the founder of modern nursing. She practiced nursing in the 19th century and came to prominence during the Crimean War, where she took care of wounded soldiers. She is credited for turning nursing care into a profession with the founding of her nursing school at St. Thomas' Hospital in London. This was the first secular nursing school in the world. Nightingale was also a prodigious and versatile writer. During her lifetime, she wrote much about nursing and medical knowledge. Those books were written in lay terms and simple English so many could understand. Even though Nightingale published this book to be used at her nursing school in England, it was meant for anyone wanting to take care of and nurse others. She discusses areas of nursing still relevant today, such as cleanliness, bedding, lighting, ventilation, and warming. Any surgeon today will tell you about the invaluable contributions nurses make to the success of a surgery. In 1907 she received the Order of Merit from the Queen of England.

Printed in an edition of three hundred copies.
Designed by Scott J. Vile at the Ascensius Press.